THE SKY IS MINE

AMY BEASHEL

ROCK THE BOAT

A Rock the Boat Book

First published by Rock the Boat,
an imprint of Oneworld Publications, 2020
Reprinted, 2020

This book contains material which some readers may find
distressing, including discussions of rape, coercive behaviour,
domestic violence and abuse. We are grateful to sexual health and
wellbeing charity Brook for undertaking a sensitivity read.

ISBN 978-1-78607-555-0 (Paperback)
ISBN 978-1-78607-864-3 (Hardback)
eISBN 978-1-78607-556-7

Typeset by Fakenham Prepress Solutions, Fakenham, Norfolk, NR21 8NL
Printed and bound in Great Britain by Clays Ltd, Elcograf S.p.A.

Oneworld Publications
10 Bloomsbury Street, London, WC1B 3SR, England
3754 Pleasant Ave, Suite 100, Minneapolis, MN 55409, USA

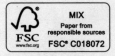

MIX
Paper from
responsible sources
FSC® C018072

For MDH, who never makes me doubt me.
And for Mum, who taught me the importance of self-worth.
In characters, yes, but so too, always, always, in me.

ONE

It's not just my breath but my voice that Jacob knocks out of me. As his palms knead hard into my chest, there are no words in my mouth, just his tongue and his 'Oh, come on, Izzy', which spreads thick and sticky as Marmite.

I hate Marmite.

And his voice? Well, it's hardly an invitation, is it? It's a right.

My body is quiet too. You'd think my skin would sizzle when he pushes my back into the heated towel rail that's ramped up so high it's hotter even than Jacob's breath and the brawl of his fingers working their way into 'Fuck, yeah, the sweet spot'. Like there's anything sweet in this. But I don't say that obviously, cos this isn't a conversation. It's a raid.

And I hate Marmite, but my body just kind of surrenders. Everything just kind of gives in.

I shouldn't be here.

Where I should be is on the other side of the bathroom door. With Grace. But Grace is with Nell, *their* bodies oozing in the pleasure they've found in each other.

''Nother drink?' he says.

But just as Jacob's hands work like cuffs around my wrists, the bathroom door opens and he's all 'Crap, Izzy', like it was me who was in charge of locking the door.

It's her. The one who's always rescued me.

'Grace!' And I'm sure I say it, that her name from my mouth is a siren so loud and so urgent that she'll run from her stumble into the sink and pull me from where I'm squished behind Jacob out into the real world, where it'll be just the two of us again.

But all my best mate does is a quick glance-over with these Prosecco-ed mutters of 'oops' and 'sorry', and then she's gone and I'm still here, still pressed into him as he reaches for the open bottle with a 'gawaaaan', as he tips vodka into my mouth, which is burning, and then I splutter alcohol into his eyes.

'Fuck's sake, Izzy,' Jacob says.

And when he pulls back and his pressure's eased, I slide down the towel rail, head like a bouncy ball on its bars, until I hit the floor and droop.

I wonder if he's gone, because Jacob's voice is kind of distant. Then he lets out this laugh that's like a puff of disgust and says something like 'gotcha' before the blast of cool air lets me know I'm still here, on the wrong side of the door, having been coaxed in by the surprise of Jacob's smile. Cos it's not like he, or anyone, has paid much attention before. And yeah, he had vodka and Coke and, call me an idiot, right, but I thought the party might be easier with a shot or two. He gave me four. All with this one-for-me-one-for-you kind of grin and those hands of his, reaching up from where he strad-dled the loo, legs spread and his groin so pleased to see me.

'I'm gonna go,' I'd said to Grace in the thirty seconds she'd spared me in the kitchen twenty minutes or so after we'd arrived.

'Noooooooooo.' And her voice was all *don't leave me* as she pulled on the sleeve of my dress like she was genuinely so keen for me to stick around that she might actually stay and talk instead of abandoning me for Nell's lips and whatever it was Nell was saying that gave Grace that brilliant glow.

But she didn't. Talk to me, I mean. And so I'd stood at the table like some kind of loser until Jacob appeared with his drink and his invitation.

I'd eyeballed Grace as I'd followed his lead into the living room, thinking if she felt it – my stare that was also a plea – she'd spot the path I was taking and freak out, cos there's no one she despises more than Jacob. And the freak-out would be a stop sign, right? But her face had been so into Nell's face that she didn't notice me leaving the room, and so I'd walked out, kind of huffy but still kind of hopeful, because Grace always comes to my rescue in the end.

'Someone sort her out, would you?' Jacob shouts to whoever in the hallway.

It might be two minutes or it might be ten before I feel a prod in my arm at the same time as 'She's totally out of it' and 'Better get Grace'. And even though I am – totally out of it, I mean – Grace doesn't come.

I message her when I'm outside. After this guy Max from my English class has lifted me to my feet and splashed my face with water. After I've walked through the living room, past the eyes and the 'oi oi's, and Jacob grunt-laughing and sniffing his fingers. When I've done that – the walk of shame, I reckon they call it – I slump against the garage door, biting back the retching, as I drunk-punch words into my phone.

Where r u?
Sorry, Iz. Nell wasn't feeling great so I'm taking her home.
But I needed u.
Sorry, so did Nell.
X
U OK, Iz?
Yes.

And it shouldn't be a surprise, not really, how easy it is for Grace to believe it. That I'm OK, I mean. But she obviously does, cos that's the last of the messages and she's probably back in Nell's arms already, while I try to keep myself upright and wonder whether or not to go home.

Thing is, there's not much choice. Even if it feels as slippery there as it did at the party, there's nowhere else to go. And maybe Mum and Daniel will be in bed. And maybe my step-dad's disapproval of the dress he said made me look like I was up for it will have passed and they'll be sleeping and the house will be as quiet as me in the bathroom with Jacob before.

'Izzy!'

Shit. Cos the vodka's in my fingers as well as my head, these stupid fumbling fingers that can't keep hold of the keys or whatever I had in my hand as a weapon on standby for when someone creeps up behind.

'Izzy!'

My feet too. These ridiculous shoes on these dumb feet that can't walk a straight line so it's no wonder he catches me, right?

'Izzy!'

And the voice is a hand, is a touch in the dark.

'Wait. I'll walk you home, yeah?'

'Max.'

'Who'd you think it was? Kylo Ren?'

'Huh?'

'Jesus, Iz. Here, let me.' And before he even says what I should let him do, there's an arm round my waist and we're walking. 'You're smashed. Seriously, you shouldn't be out on your own.'

If I were Grace, I'd have an answer for that. But I'm not Grace, am I? I'm pissed.

And I'm guessing Max must have brought me back before disappearing into the night, because, like magic, I'm home.

'What time do you call this?'

I swear I nearly crap myself when a voice comes like a burglar alarm out of the dark.

I can see the shape of him on the floor, leaning against the wall under a framed page from a book about feelings Mum bought me when I was a kid. *Happiness*, it says, but when I flick the switch for the light, Daniel looks so far from happiness the irony's not even funny.

'What are you like, eh, Isabel?'

And maybe with the vodka I misread his face, cos even though it's nothing like happy, his voice is different from the disgusted sneer when I left for the party earlier. None of the anger or disappointment. Softer maybe, like my stepdad might actually give a toss if I'm feeling awful, like really awful, like he did when we hadn't known him long and I fell from my bike, and before the tears even had a chance to hit my cheeks, he'd scooped up the heap of me and smothered me with kisses he said were from fairies who'd given him powers to make me well. And, sure, I already knew fairies weren't real but, as with everything else he said, I believed him.

'Come here,' he says now, a whole foot taller than me so his chin rests on my head when he brings me to his chest and tells me he has concerns. And it all feels kind of weird when he says he's worried about boys, you know, because I've obviously been drinking, and then there's that up-for-it dress, and I need to be more careful because 'You're so special', and it's not just his hand on my back, but his finger. And yeah, that's attached to his hand, but one finger has a different kind of touch.

Mum appears at the top of the stairs and his hand flattens into a palm.

'You OK, Isabel?' Her voice tries to be a glass half full.

'She's good,' Daniel says before I can say anything, using the bulk of him to shift me out of her sight.

And I guess from how her footsteps take her back into the bedroom, like Grace, Mum must also be choosing to believe that I'm fine.

TWO

It's not the first time someone's slipped me a pair of inflated tits under the table. And even though Miss Green's on to him, I'm pretty sure it won't be the last time Jacob pulls up some hardcore on his phone and passes it round the class like a tin of Quality Street at Christmas.

And if it weren't for his juiced-up excitement, I could hand it straight back, but there's this film of sweat from Jacob's palms, and what with that and the shock of that mesh of bodies going at it like hairless animals in a screen-sized cage in a zoo, the phone falls to the floor in an all-eyes-on-me kind of clatter, and Jacob rolls his eyes, like, *seriously, Izzy*, as if I'm the idiot here.

It's stupid really, how I can look at the phone as I pick it up but not at Jacob as I put it down on the desk, how his hard stare makes me feel as naked as those women in the film.

'Honestly, you lot –' Miss Green doesn't clock Callum Gun's hands miming just what he'd like to do to her bum as she walks from the whiteboard towards me – 'how many times have you been told? No phones in class.'

'Sorry, miss.' Though Jacob's voice is a sorry-not-sorry kind of smirk as Miss Green picks it up, turns it over and sees the mass of skin, the wet mouths and the perfectly timed shot of the man getting just what he came for. 'I'll delete it, miss,' he says, but we all know that if he does, there are a thousand more where that came from – those films he called 'life lessons' when I saw him watching one on the bus a few months back and he did that V shape with his fingers, tongue between them, the other boys sniggering and, yeah, some of the girls too. 'Come on, miss,' he says now, 'it's a laugh, innit.'

But Miss Green, the inside of her bottom lip pulled back between her teeth, doesn't look like she thinks that's true.

'Don't be a prude, miss. It's just bodies.' He winks. 'Natural, innit.'

I catch Grace's eye, like, *say something*.

'Ask Izzy, miss,' Jacob mutters.

I swear my face melts into my body, melts into the floor.

Only it doesn't, not really. There's too much of me, too many inches of thick shame to disappear, and though Grace's hand on my thigh is an anchor, it's not enough to steady the shake, which starts in my fingers but spreads like gossip through the college corridors to the rest of me, cos though the click of Miss Green's heels on the floor might have prevented her from hearing Jacob's jibe about me, the rest of the class received it loud and clear.

Not that it's anything new. Because, no kidding, it's five weeks since that party, and Jacob's still getting off on how easily I shrivel when he's around.

'Watch yourself, Mansfield.'

If Jacob's voice was a *sorry, not sorry*, Grace's is a *you will be*. But his shoulders are, like, *whatever*, as he stands, all that six foot two of him, following Miss Green to the front of the classroom, where he leans over her desk and in that voice,

8

deep as hell since three or so years ago when he and his mates hulked from boy body to man body, he apologises, just sincere enough this time.

Miss Green tells him, 'Any more of that and, honestly, Jacob, I'll have no choice.'

'Thanks, miss,' he says, head down as he turns away from her, slipping the phone into his pocket, where he makes a pantomime grab of his dick. He mouths in my direction, 'You love it.'

Max Dale shakes his head, like, *you nob, Mansfield*.

But he's smiling.

Everyone's smiling, right, cos it's natural, innit? Anything else, and you're just a prude.

THREE

'All I'm *saying* is: I'm so *totally* glad boys aren't *my* thing, that's all.' Grace's voice is, like, totally am-dram. Ever since Mrs James, our Year Three teacher, told her how wonderfully she used emphasis after her turn reading *Fantastic Mr Fox* aloud in class, she's been sure to verbally underline at least one word per sentence. 'Jacob Mansfield is *such* a *creep*.'

She reckoned the breeze along the seafront would shift the humiliation that's smeared like cheap sun cream across my skin, but the June heat's making me stickier, which fits with the indignity, I guess; at least there's no doubting that I now look as crap as I feel.

As usual, Grace glides through, talking at a hundred miles an hour, unaffected by humidity or shame. 'If I was *straight* and had to choose from that *bunch of pervs*, I swear I'd die. *Literally*,' she says, and, not for the first time, I wish I was gay too, because my best mate has a point – they don't make it easy, those boys, and if I *were* gay, maybe Grace wouldn't need Nell.

'*Nell* would *never* be like that,' she says.

And in my head, I'm thinking, *Yeah, yeah, we all know Nell would never be like that, cos Nell is never anything but perfect, right?*

'OMG, Izzy, it's *bliss*!' Grace had swooned when, six weeks into their relationship, they'd 'taken the plunge' and spent a night in a Margate B & B, looking the following morning like two flushed explorers who've discovered a new moon.

'Taken the plunge?' I said, as we drank hot chocolate after, partly to dissect and partly so she wouldn't be entirely lying when she told her mum she'd been hanging with me in the Old Town. 'It sounds so wet.'

And she smiled, like, *yeah, that's the point,* and though she was holding my hand at the time, like she always does when we're revealing secrets, I felt this thin line being drawn between us, and I've had no hope of finding my way back to her side since.

'Max isn't so bad.' I look away from Grace to the wind farm as I say it, or whisper it really, because I know what Grace will say. She'll say, in a voice that sounds like one of those feminist books she's always taking from the library, that I deserve better and nothing is better than something if the something thinks jacking off to that misogynistic smut is OK.

'Yeah, not so bad if you *like* to spend time with someone whose idea of romance is sending out a group Snapchat asking *three* fingers or *four.*'

I know she's proving some political point, but you'd think that, over a month on, Grace would stop using the most mortifying moment of my life to do it.

'That was Jacob,' I say, like it matters, cos right from the beginning, when we first started college and Jacob made some comment about us being scissor sisters, Grace lumped all that lot together in a box labelled 'scum'. 'Max is actually quite sweet.' And I think of how he made sure I got home safely from *that* party and how, last Friday, when Grace was off with

Nell – when isn't she off with Nell? – and Max was at McDonald's, he called out my name as I took my chocolate thick shake and asked if I wanted to walk home.

Normally, I'd have been, like, *hold on*, and disappeared to the loo to call Grace and ask what she thought, but Grace's giggles at lunchtime had made it pretty clear what she and Nell were up to that night, so, without saying yes or no, I just shrugged and fell in step alongside him, realising quick enough how even Max's voice had less swagger when Jacob Mansfield wasn't in tow.

'What you listening to?' Max could have just pointed at the earphones hanging round my neck, but he actually lifted one from my shoulder and nodded at the phone poking out from the pocket of my bag. 'Play it,' he said.

If I'd put it like this to Grace, I swear she'd have been rolling her eyes, like, *you just don't get it, do you, Izzy?*, and citing it as an example of Max's *patriarchal power*. But it was more gentle than that, more of a question, and not even a piss-take when I had to explain it wasn't Radio 1 or Spotify but this show, *Desert Island Discs,* that basically sums up my childhood with Mum.

'It's a radio programme,' I said to Max. 'On Radio 4.'

'Radio 4! Isn't that for old people?!'

'Not always!'

And I reached for the earphones, but Max was all 'I'm kidding, Izzy!' and totally 'Go on then, tell me more…'

'It's simple really. Each guest imagines they're cast away to an island and has to choose the music they'd take with them.' Funny, isn't it, how easily the words came when it was just the two of us. 'Eight songs. Possibly the only music they'll have for the rest of their lives!'

'Cool.'

And I couldn't tell if Max was serious, but: 'It is!' I was practically gushing. 'Cool, I mean.' Though really it's so much more.

I've been listening to them all again, those *Desert Island Discs*. On my own this time around, although sometimes, but not so much recently, if Daniel's out I'll give Mum an earphone, and while it's not the green chair the two of us would squish into when I was a kid – that didn't go with Daniel's leather sofas apparently – the shared wires bring us close enough for me to feel her shoulders drop and her breaths deepen, for me to believe she's also remembering how *Desert Island Discs* was once our thing.

Because it was definitely *a thing*. We'd kick off Sundays listening to pop music in a super deep bath. She'd let me wash her hair, stick a flannel to her face and make shampoo potions, which I'd rub into the purplish lines on her tummy, and we'd marvel at my wizard genius as, over time, they faded silver. When the water was cold and we were wrinkled, we'd get dressed, and I'd curl into Mum's lap in that charity-shop green chair she bartered down to seven pounds fifty-five after we first moved out of Great-grandma's place. And she'd stretch to switch from Radio 1 to Radio 4, ready to welcome guest after guest on to this island we'd made perfect for two.

And my mates reckon it's a bit weird cos, I know, right, *Desert Island Discs* isn't exactly *Teletubbies* or *Postman Pat*. And, to be clear, I *did* watch those things too. But Sundays were special. 'Incredible', Mum would say sometimes when the castaway had chosen their eight tracks, their luxury and their book, struggling occasionally to decide which one record they'd save if their collection was at risk of being lost to the sea, 'what some people do with their lives…' She'd hold me for some time after. 'What they overcome.'

And last Friday, Max's smile when I did hit *play* – it was curious, none of that sneering they're so full of in the canteen. And it felt kind of nice, kind of all right, to be with Max Dale when Grace was so obviously caught up in Nell.

''S cool.' He nodded, like, *honestly, Iz, I'm not taking the piss*, returning the earphone when the castaway's track ended.

Jacob was hurling 'oi oi's from across the street by then, sniffing and waving his fingers, and it was clear the moment was done.

'Later!' Max was away, over the road, shrugging off whatever Jacob was saying, with one last look back at me before they were gone.

'Quite *sweet*?' Grace says now. 'This *flake* is sweet, Iz.' She licks at the 99. 'Max Dale is *not* sweet. He might not be as gross as Jacob, but he's *best mates* with the guy, and that's got to say *something*.'

'I'm best mates with *you*. I hope people don't judge me for that!'

I take a swipe at her ice cream, but she's too quick.

'Should have got your own,' she says. Then, like always, she says, 'Have a bit if you want.' But I'm on this food plan my stepdad Daniel's cooked up for my mum and me. 'Suit yourse— Oh, hold it a mo, would you?' And the Mr Whippy's practically in my face as she starts digging for her ringing phone in her bag. 'Babe,' she says, as the cold slips down my throat and into my belly. 'Sure,' she says, 'about ten minutes, yeah?'

And the cold mixes with the sad cos it's clear I'm about to be abandoned. It's practically a habit now, how Grace leaves me for Nell. Even the chocolate's no consolation.

'You don't mind, do you, Iz?'

Of course I shake my head, *no, I don't mind*, because as much as I hate that face Grace has whenever she hears from her girlfriend – that wide-eyed look of the Beast in the animated version when he meets Beauty on the stairs for a dance, sporting a suit and that crazy big can't-believe-his-luck kind of grin – it offers me hope, too. Hope, I guess, that for all the crappy places it can take you, it's also possible love will lead you to that top-step moment when anything seems possible, when the Beast changes from a monster and a happily ever after doesn't seem so much of a fairy-tale trick after all.

'Go! Have fun.' I mean it too.

Just like I mean the smile as she skips off and mean it still as Max Dale appears from behind a beach hut, asking in that not-so-swagger kind of voice if I fancy meeting up later. Grinning, totally friendly, totally cool, he says, 'Thought maybe you've got some more old-people radio shows you wanna share?'

FOUR

'Who was he?' Daniel's voice is a can of Coke – I know the rising bubbles are in there but can't be sure how fierce they'll be until he opens the can. It's always tricky to tell how much he's been shaken.

'Who do you mea—'

But my stepdad's speaking over me, already on his next lot of questions, asking if 'that boy' goes to my college and where did we head to looking so close and so conspiratorial.

'Imagine my surprise,' he says, stirring milk into the tea he's making for me, taking the sugar from the cupboard but with a quick glance at my belly, an almost undetectable shake of his head, putting it back without adding any, and then arranging three cookies on a plate and leaving them on the end of the breakfast bar, just within arm's reach. 'I wasn't sure if it was you at first. I didn't think you were the kind of girl to be out with a boy on your own.'

He takes a biscuit, delicate bites, elongated chews, eyes on me while my gaze flits from him to the plate, where a chocolate chip has come loose.

It's just a chocolate chip. But it's not, not really. It's will-power. Or, on Daniel's part, just power, full stop.

Daniel's behind me then, his breath in my ear. 'There's certainly no mistaking you from behind though, is there,

Isabel,' he says, the smile in his voice as cool as his hand on my back, that flesh between my T-shirt and jeans. Two of his fingertips press and pull on my skin until Mum appears, and he sweeps his palm away, like it was never there, to her waist, easing her from the two remaining cookies. 'Nah-ah-ah! Not on the food plan, remember!' And he slides the plate along the work surface straight past me and across to the other side, scooting around to catch it before it falls. 'Save!'

I don't know if it's the actor in him, but Daniel's always saving things: biscuits, the day, us. I swear he's waiting for a part as a knight just so he can come home in the shining armour. As if looking like George Clooney isn't enough. He'd opt for the white horse too, come charging in like he always does with his facial-ed skin, his massaged cuticles and his dyed grey hair to cast his net across the room, hauling Mum in with those practised lines of his, not the ones from scripts but from the part of Daniel that personally wrote their wedding vows in which he promised to love her fully, endlessly, differently from the way anyone has loved her before.

'He's passionate,' Mum's said in the past, and my mates would back her up, swooning like they do when he dons the tux with the undone bow tie, suit jacket hooked on his finger and slung over his shoulder in what appears to be a casual way but, believe me, I've seen him rehearsing it in the mirror before heading off to some party so middle-aged women can have their photo taken with their arms wrapped around a fake George.

So my stepdad isn't some horsebacked prince but a look-alike, though he prefers to tell everyone he's an actor really, the

George thing is just for fun, but with Clooney being so popular, '*and* so handsome', Daniel jokes in that way that manages to be self-deprecating even though he's basically saying he's, like, really hot, the celebrity-double work just keeps on coming so 'it'd be foolish to say no'. Daniel is anything but foolish.

'Come on then, Isabel, spill the beans.' He winks at Mum. 'I believe our little minx here may have bagged her first boyfriend.'

'He's *not* my boyfriend.'

'The lady doth protest too much.' Crumbs from the second cookie spill from between his teeth.

'He's just a friend.'

Grace would kill me for even calling Max that. For even walking those few minutes with Max and shrugging my shoulders, like, *yeah*, when he asked if I was free later.

'All I'm saying is I hope you don't do anything you shouldn't with your *friend*.'

What I want most is to snap Daniel's fingers in half as he makes those air quotes around 'friend', but I don't, obviously, cos if Mum's anything to go by, the best thing to do is just ignore the fact that Daniel's being a complete and utter dick and just sit there staring at that one last cookie like it might actually be the answer to your woes.

As if.

She won't even look at me. Picks at her bitten nails instead, pushing them into her hairline, where the red, which looked so electric in those photos she'd begged her grandmother to take of the two of us when I was a baby, is now muted by thicker, wirier stands of grey.

'You wouldn't want to end up like Vicky Pollard here, would you?' He nudges Mum with his elbow.

My face must be, like, *I don't get it*.

'Teenage mum,' Daniel says. 'What a slaaaaaaaaaag.' His voice has echoes of a TV-show insult – a comedy, right. A joke? But Mum had enough of that at the time, I reckon.

I get it at college too. Boys spitting the word out in fake coughs as I walk down the corridor. The girls don't bother with names, but their quick-up-and-down-on-me eyes are as lethal as slurs, and then there are their giggles behind hands, which have probably been in way worse places than mine are rumoured to have gone at that party.

Ugh, that party. Too much vodka and not enough dinner or Grace, and I couldn't stop Jacob Mansfield doing whatever he did in that bathroom. The rest would have been a blur if it weren't for the picture he took of me slumped into the wall, my up-for-it dress ridden over my thighs, legs slightly apart and mouth dropped open like he'd literally only just pulled out his tongue. *Three fingers or four*, he scrawled in red across my body in the photo, sending it to his mates, who sent it to their mates, who sent it to their mates, cos obviously it was, like, the funniest thing ever.

You know, someone once said how the things that aren't great at the time are the things that will eventually become your best stories to tell in the pub. Dark humour maybe. So perhaps there's hope, right, that, one day, I will tell the tale of Jacob Mansfield and his fingers out loud and it won't feel like fire in my bones.

Today's not forever, right? Things can change.

'I'm just teasing, Isabel.' Daniel's voice is a don't-be-a-baby-now kind of chiding. 'Joking aside, you should be careful though. Shouldn't she, Stephanie?'

Mum looks at him, like, *whatever you say, Daniel*.

'You want to save yourself for someone special,' he says, not for the first time but for the first time in front of my mum. 'Not like your mother here, sleeping with any Tom, Dick or Harry when she was sixteen.'

I swear her face doesn't even flicker. My heart, on the other hand – my heart is raging. Because they may have been young, but Mum's promised me my dad was special. She doesn't say this now though, does she? Just sits there as Daniel takes his time chewing that last bloody cookie.

'Oops, sorry,' he says, hand over his mouth in Oscar-worthy shock at his greed. 'I didn't even offer you one. Probably for the best though, eh.' Mum's as blank as ever when he pinches her bum. 'We all know what you ladies are like: a moment on the lips, forever on the hips. I'll make us something healthy for dinner while you do your homework, shall I?'

Only I don't do my homework. What I do is sit with my Jar of Sunshine, taking off its lid, removing the yellow beads my real dad gave me and rolling them between my fingers before tucking them back inside along with these whispers about how special he was. How different he was. How much I wish he was here.

And then I think about calling Grace. And then I sit and think about Grace with Nell. And then I sit and think about Grace with Nell and me with nobody, until my phone beeps with a message from Max Dale saying he meant what he said earlier, about meeting up, and, sure, Grace says a nobody is better than a somebody if the somebody isn't the right body, but she's not the one sitting on her own, desperate to avoid dinner and its inevitable scene.

Sure, I say to Max, a small part of my big body wondering if there's some trick in his offer.

This isn't a joke, is it? I ask him.

And he's straight back with a *No, promise.*

So, before I have time to doubt the decision, I put my Jar of Sunshine back on the shelf, and I go.

FIVE

'I've been working on the music I'd take,' Max says.

I must look at him like, *huh?*

'To my island, Izzy! It's hard, man. To narrow it down to eight. Didn't you say they can take a book too?'

'Yeah' is all I can manage. I want to be funny. I want to be cool. Basically, I want to be Grace.

'Go on then.' Max nudges me with his knee as he hands me a Freddo with one hand and picks up a pebble with the other. 'What would yours be?'

And I wonder about that feelings book mum bought me, about taking the *happiness* Daniel cut out of it and sticking it back in, because maybe with that and the desert-island isolation I'd have a chance of finally putting all my screwed-up feelings straight. But no way I'm admitting that to Max, obviously, so: 'I dunno. Carol Ann Duffy?'

'Carol Ann Duffy?' Max's voice is all *are you sure?*, and I'm convinced he'll do a Jacob and call her a dyke, but: 'You mean the poet?'

'Yeah, we read her in English Lit.'

'I know.'

Of course he does – he was there, wasn't he? Slouched beside Jacob, who was sly-winking: 'That Duffy, she's one of your lot, isn't she, Grace? Go for her, would you? I mean, you like a white one, don't you? Saw you at that party and you was well into that bird. Whatsherface? Nell, isn't it?' And it was all kinds of spineless, but I couldn't deny the relief that for once they were talking about *that* party and hadn't yet mentioned Jacob's fingers or me. 'Don't your mum and dad mind their little black princess going out with a white girl?'

'White girl, black girl...so long as it's not a little nob like you, Jacob, they don't really care.'

She always has the answer, does Grace.

'"Anon", that's one of Duffy's poems, right?'

And I don't know what to say now, because Max Dale talking about poetry is as much of a shock as Max Dale inviting me out, as Max Dale not laughing, like, *fooled you*, when I met him by Tesco Express, half expecting Jacob to appear from behind the bins to take another photo of just what an idiot I am for actually believing Max Dale might want to spend time with me. But the thing is, he does. Want to spend some time with me, I mean, cos he was all smiles and 'All right, Izzy', totally shy even as he suggested we go to the beach.

And now, with his Freddos and his pebbles, he looks at me like, *come on then, you're the one who kicked this game off.*

'Yeah, I like that one, "Anon". Depressing though.'

Max looks at me like, *how come?*

'Women not having a voice and all that.'

'Different these days though, innit?' Max says. 'Look at Grace. No one can say *she* hasn't got a voice.' And *his* voice? He tries to make it as cool as his Coke but, like the can in the evening sunshine, it can't quite stay chilled. 'Speaking of Grace –' he plonks the whole bag of Freddos in my lap – 'I know she's got a girlfriend, Izzy, but do you reckon that it might just be, you know, a phase?'

And thank god for Max's nerves because all those jitters with his fingers and the pebbles and the looking at me, like, *don't tell her I've said this* – yeah, it all adds up to him not picking up on my disappointment.

'You like Grace?' I ask him, and he nods, shy but not quite defeated.

'Yeah. Well, sort of.' He just about dares to look up. 'And I get she's gay, but Jacob reckons all girls come round in the end.'

And I might not say anything, but the rolling eyes must convey exactly what I think of Jacob's theory because Max shakes his head, like, *all right, point taken.*

'Did it look like a phase when you saw her at that party with her girlfriend?'

'S'pose,' he says. 'I'm surprised you can even remember.'

Honestly, I'd rather he swooned over Grace than we talk about *that*.

'You were gone, Izzy.'

'No more than you or Jacob or any of your other mates.'

'Isn't the same for us though, is it?'

And I wonder how much Max would like Grace if she were here now, laying into him for that.

'You fancy getting something to eat?' he says.

'Haven't we already?' I hold up the Freddos in my lap, like, *what more could we possibly need?*

Max is all *fair point*, when there are these shouts from up by the huts.

'Eh, eh, what's going on here then, Maxy? Getting yourself a bit of Izzy action, are you?'

Jacob's not looking at his mate though. His eyes are on me.

'Loosened you up a bit, didn't I, Fingers?'

Despite our silence, he keeps going.

'You need to drop her back at KFC, Max. Recycle her bucket.'

My big toe finds a small patch of sand among the pebbles, digs in.

'You at football in the morning?' Max asks.

I see what Max is doing, but changing the subject doesn't stop the burn in my face, that churn in the pit of my belly.

'Yeah, mate.'

The two of them drift up the path in a rush of banter and brawn, and I wonder how long it'll last, this easy chat about my vagina. It's not like either of them is calling it that but, let's face it, that's what it comes down to. What I boil down to. For them.

'Sorry 'bout Jacob,' Max says when he comes back, snatching the last Freddo from my palm. 'He's all right really. He's only trying to be funny.'

And I'd love to believe him but...'Is it though?'

'What?'

'Is it funny?'

You'd think from his silence that I'd asked Max the square root of 3.8 billion.

'What Jacob says, I mean. What he does. Is it actually funny?'

And I'm not usually one for confrontation. I mean, there's

no way I'd speak with Jacob like this, but Max isn't Jacob. It's not that I know what Max is exactly, but he's not that.

'Like the other day, when he was banging on about the fingers thing for, like, the millionth time, you know, when he said he knows how much I liked his sweet stuff.'

'Oh, yeah, with the Curly Wurly.' And maybe it *is* actually funny, because then Max is kind of laughing when he remembers how Jacob unwrapped the long chocolate bar, poking it up inside my T-shirt, prodding my boobs with it, playing to the crowd, asking if anyone fancied fetching the crumbs. 'It's not like he actually touched you though, Izzy.'

And yeah, there were no fingers that time, I guess.

'Shall we then?'

My eyebrows must be, like, *what?*

'Get something to eat?' Max says, smiling as if *'it's not like he actually touched you'* will have undone all the shame that comes with Jacob's 'jokes'.

'Sure,' I tell him. Cos it's not like it's his fault Jacob's a complete bellend. And, more importantly, it's not like I've got anything better to do, what with Grace otherwise engaged and my stepdad on the prowl at home.

So we start walking up to McDonald's and Max turns to me, totally serious, and tells me, 'Your old-person programme's not so bad, you know.'

'My old-person programme? I hope you're not demeaning the iconic brilliance that is *Desert Island Discs*?'

'Not demeaning it at all actually. I quite liked it.'

'You listened to it?'

'Yep. Some comedian. He only went and admitted he was

a virgin until he was twenty-six! Twenty-six!' Max repeats, with a quick look over his shoulder to check no one but me is listening. 'No way I'm waiting that long.'

'So you're…'

'Yeah.' His voice is a finger to his mouth, like, *don't say anything though.*

'The way you and Jacob and that lot bang on…'

'Just bants though, innit.'

Yeah, right, isn't it always? But I don't say that, obviously, because I'm not Grace, am I? Never will be.

'Sorry,' I say, when we're done with the Happy Meal and back outside in the late-evening sun. Max looks at me, like, *what for?*

'About Grace.'

'Whatever.' And if Max's voice were a pair of glasses, they'd be rose-tinted to match his not-totally-given-up-yet grin.

'Max.'

He turns around when I call him back.

'You reckon you could have a word with Jacob? See if he'll ease up on all that finger stuff?'

'Sure,' he says, 'but you do know it's just ban—'

I put my earphones in as hard as they'll possibly go so I don't have to hear any more.

SIX

'You smell like fast food.'

I should have thought of the stink of it. Of Daniel's hound-like nose and his face when he spots that I've strayed from his plan to save my arse from its meteoric proportions. His words, not mine.

'Like mother like daughter,' he says, and he's all smiles, right, but the shake of his head's a different story – the one that ends with him pointing at those pictures of models he's pinned to the fridge as 'thinspiration' and me looking at my thighs in the mirror wondering how all those other girls do it. Fall out of hate with their bodies, I mean.

'You're beautiful,' Mum whispers when Daniel leaves the kitchen, but her voice is too much like tissue paper to wrap me up in anything that feels like safety or strength or truth. I wish she'd say it when he was here. So the all-rightness of my fat doesn't come across as an afterthought or some secret she's so obviously ashamed of.

'That your boyfriend?' Daniel calls from the other room when my phone beeps with a message, and he laughs this laugh that's totally not funny, but Mum still gives me this look, like, *well?* Like she actually believes Daniel might be on to something. But even if Max were my boyfriend, which obviously he isn't, it's not him cos the number's a new one, the words 'photo' and 'frigid' flashing on my screen like the red man, like *do not cross*, but sometimes something pushes you into the oncoming traffic and you go.

'Isabel!' But Daniel's fuss about my elephant gallop up the stairs is the least of my worries because the mystery sender's got to be Jacob and his words are a ten-tonne truck.

I have another photo. Shows your not so frigid side. Meet me to work something out.

Jacob?

You recognised me. Nice.

What photo?

For me to know and you to avoid. My house. Tonight. ASAP. Or Fingers XL goes viral.

Shit. Like, proper shit. Like heart-in-the-mouth, I-could-die-here shit. And maybe Max was right when he said I was gone at that party. Because my body may have been there, but that bit of my brain that should have stored whatever it was that happened with Jacob was too drenched in vodka to make any pictures of its own. To make any memories that might have given me some kind of clue what Jacob has on me. What Jacob did to me. When I was gone.

Think of the desert island, Izzy.

Because sometimes it helps, right? To imagine there is nothing but me and the sand and the sea. To think what happens to me in my world is my own doing, to think I can choose my narrative as easily as I can choose my songs. All fine in theory, but what if I can't? What if some dickhead from my college takes my narrative and slaps photos over it, the way Grace and I used to cover our notebooks in Years Seven and

Eight, when it was still OK to stick photos of Harry Styles on everything, a way of making the workbook more enticing. Only Jacob's photos are gonna make everything so much worse. What happens then? When I'm trapped in the story of the Finger Slag and someone else is dictating my ending?

'Mum and Dad've gone out.' Jacob quickly checks the street and I'm not sure if he's looking for last-minute signs of his parents or for anyone who may have clocked him going in with Izzy Chambers. 'We have plenty of time,' he says, and his voice is a *know what I mean?* and his hands are a guide dog leading me blindly up the staircase and into his room.

'Sorry 'bout the mess.'

No kidding, cos it's the kind of shitstorm of clothes and books and crisp packets that'd send Daniel into full-on thunder.

''S all right,' I say, even though none of it is – all right, I mean. Not the mess, not the being here, not the rustle in my head that says *run*, not the weight in my legs that stops me.

Then Jacob shifts his copy of *Men's Health* to make space on the bed and pats the duvet like you'd pat a dog, like all this is sweet really, you know, in spite of what he said just now about this photo he has of me and his fingers and my…well, you get the picture.

'Your face is in it too,' he'd said, like that was such a good thing. 'You were well up for it.'

And I'd have asked for the evidence, but his hands were already on my back, telling me exactly what I'd need to do to keep that picture between the two of us.

'You don't mind, do you, Izzy...' he says now, and there's this flicker of a moment, as he shifts from the mattress, and I think this was all his idea of a sick trick, and relief floods into me like the Jack Daniel's rushing from the bottle into Jacob's glass, 'if I put something on to get us in the mood, yeah?'

And the laptop screen's not big but it's like IMAX the way it fills the room with its full-on tits and arse, and those two girls to the one guy are nothing, nothing, *nothing* like me, which is the point, I guess.

And I should say something, but Jacob's kisses are harder now and his tongue – it's like the underside of satsuma peel, furred by the Jack Daniel's and Coke he's knocked back with the two bags of Monster Munch since I got here. The empty packets scrunch between the sheet and the skin of my back when he lies me down. And his fingers, probably still coated in Monster dust, claw at my folds as I suggest that, maybe, I'll go.

'You can't leave,' Jacob says, winking as he points to the crotch of his jeans stretched tight like he's part Hulk and he isn't to blame for what might happen when it bursts through.

And I know what they say, a man thinks with his dick, but I'm not sure that's true, cos his dick doesn't look like it's thinking at all. If anything, it looks like it's up for a fight.

'We had a deal,' he says.

And his hands too are bulging, or the veins of them, gripped tight on my shoulders, knuckles as yellow-white as Monsters, scored with fine lines the colour of rare steak the way Daniel has it so it bleeds on to his peas. You'd think Jacob's fingers would be easier to look at than that bulldozer

31

dick, but this view's no kinder, his lockjaw-hold making a concertina of my flesh, his smile detached from the clench he has on me and his eyes twinkling as if he's Santa Claus about to make all my Christmas dreams come true.

From what Grace told me, sex is like magic. It makes you like that woman who steps into the box and disappears to this other place, where only one other person in the whole entire world knows you're there. Because they're the one that sent you.

I'd disappear if I could, but I can't.

'I should go,' I say, but my words are an echo and his room is a cave with its closed curtains and the bedside lamp suddenly switched off by his swift fingers, which somehow turn to fire in the dark, spreading wild across my body so I can no longer tell which bit of him is where because the whole of Jacob is on me, against me, burning itself into me as my echo presses into what might be his chest but could be his shoulder. Whatever piece of him is so close to my mouth, it melts my ability to speak, any words I try to summon seeping into a wet patch of nothing on his shirt.

'You like that, huh?' Jacob says, cos maybe my damp echo wadded with his collar or his sleeve sounds like pleasure. 'Izzy Chambers,' he says, and his voice isn't mean. It's just somewhere else, in the film on his computer maybe, with those girls who are all 'yes's and groans and loving whatever it is the man does to them.

I hate him. Him and all those words he's drawling into boa constrictor shapes around me, and his eyes as heavy a weight upon my chest as his hands.

'Let's get a picture.' One of his hands comes away from my hip to snatch his phone. 'Cheeeeeeeese,' he says, like his bed is a monument, like we're tourists, or friends.

And he's laughing, but this is no joke. Because here I am now, on Jacob Mansfield's monument bed, with Jacob Mansfield undoing my flies, fingers digging at my knickers like he's playing Tetris and flipping shapes to fit them in a hole, those Monster knuckles inflicting tiny punches against my pubic bone, which kind of shrinks back into me, as I tell Jacob Mansfield's chest or shoulder, 'Wait.' Only Jacob Mansfield's chest or shoulder isn't listening, cos Jacob Mansfield's mouth is making these other noises, these grunts like the howler monkeys we heard when Daniel took Mum and me on our first 'family date' to the zoo.

'Izzy Chambers,' Jacob repeats now, and I wonder if, like me, he can't quite believe that I'm here.

Isn't this what I wanted? A boy and his hands and his mouth saying my name?

'You OK, yeah?'

I must have known this was what I was coming for, right? When I climbed up the stairs of Jacob's house and into his bedroom with the door pushed to? When I sat on the bed while he ate his Monster Munch? When I shook my head no to the crisps and said nothing when he kissed me? Isn't this what I expected when Jacob pushed me gently on to the pillow and reminded me of our deal?

'Izzy,' Jacob says.

And I wonder if this is it, if this is the moment when he'll offer to stop so I don't have to come up with a yes or a no, but all he says, as he slips the condom from the packet with these fingers so delicate you'd think he actually cares, is: 'Don't say I don't look out for you, yeah? You ready?'

But before I can answer, Jacob Mansfield has taken my virginity as easily as he took that photo with his phone.

SEVEN

There was this book Mum got me about feelings when I was a kid. She was paranoid, I reckon, that I was gonna be messed up, by not having a dad maybe, or the fact that my grandparents still refused to acknowledge that I was around. She didn't come right out and say it and obviously she tried to sweep all that bad stuff under the carpet, but kids aren't stupid, right? No matter how thick the surface, they feel the bumps in things. I could read it on Mum's face, when we'd write her parents a Christmas card each year, and she'd lift the post off the mat on those Advent mornings, how the pain she felt at their lack of reply was like treading on Lego bricks. It eased off after Daniel came – he filled a hole, I guess, told us it was their loss and we didn't need them anyway. 'Just the three of us,' he'd say, and we'd huddle in, welcoming the barrier he was shaping against the outside world and gratefully edging in.

The feelings book had come before then, when it was Mum perhaps who needed the reassurance, when she'd pause on the page that described loneliness, hug me a little tighter and then later, when she thought I was sleeping, whisper to her friends, who were finishing uni by then or moving in with their boyfriends and forging careers, plus all that other stuff 'normal twenty-somethings' do. And though she'd have died a little if she'd known she was letting me in on her secret, it was clear *I* was the thing that separated her from normal, that the catch of being sixteen and pregnant didn't stop with her giving birth. So I was her hangover, I s'pose. Not the kind her mates had – theirs were a day at most – whereas Mum has been stuck with me for a lifetime. I looked at the book, but that mix of regret and shame I was feeling, not for anything I'd done, just for living – well, there was no page for that.

Mum seemed less bothered by what the normals were doing once she met Daniel. And that, along with all the other benefits of their relationship – a bigger bedroom, a brides-maid's dress, a holiday once a year – made me love him like crazy too because I could really believe Mum didn't love *me* less for everything I'd stolen from her. It was Daniel's idea to cut the *happiness* from the book and frame it, hang it on the wall so it was the first thing we saw when we got in.

So obviously that's what I see now, when I come home from whatever just happened with Jacob, already wondering what it is that I'm feeling, whether it's relief that it's done or just a big fat sack of shame. I don't know where the rest of the book's got to, all those other pages like 'sadness' and 'confu-sion' and 'guilt'. We weren't expecting any of those once we had Daniel so we had no need to keep them, I guess, but I tip my room over anyway, hoping maybe I'll find them and pin them to my T-shirt so they might seep into me, make me feel *something*, which has got to be better than the blank page I turned into once Jacob was done with me.

'That was all right, wasn't it, Izzy?' he'd said after, more of a *you can be off now then* than an actual enquiry into how I'd found it. Whatever *it* was.

And he'd just shrugged his shoulders, like, *what?*, when I started to cry and kind of mumbled it wasn't him, it was me.

But was it? Me, I mean? Or was it him? Or the two of us? Or something else I don't have a name for?

Whatever it was, I wanted my mum. Pathetic, right? But I wanted her to be there when I got home, acting like some normal paranoid parent who thinks her daughter might be up to no good. Waiting up for me because I hadn't told her where I was going and it was dark outside and she was worried. '*What is it?*' she'd say, this imaginary mother of mine. '*You can tell me,*' she'd say. '*I just want to help you. To protect you.*' And she would.

But she wasn't and she didn't and she won't. Because she's sleeping. Keeping the ten o'clock bedtime Daniel insists she needs for her beauty sleep, cos it's so obvious, right, how Daniel's rules are so much more important than me.

I change into my pyjamas. Could I burn the clothes? The knickers I've balled with the rest of them shoved beneath my bed because I swear I can smell it, that whatever it was that just happened is stuck in the fabric, not just of the underwear and jeans and T-shirt but of me. What I need is a wash, a scrub, a way to grow new and untouched skin. But a shower would be too loud, too risky, so I make do with changing into my pyjamas and am climbing into bed when —

'Izzy! *Izzy!*'

Jacob.

I hadn't realised quite how much I never wanted to hear him say my name again. But he's here. Saying it. And not quietly either. When I open my bedroom window, he looks

37

up, grinning like those boys in Hollywood movies who've thrown stones to get their wannabe girlfriend's attention.

'How do you even know where I liv—'

'Max. Walked you home, didn't he? The night of the,' Jacob wiggles his fingers, grins.

'Please.' My eyes flit from him to the crack between my door and the carpet, willing it to stay black, because light would mean movement would mean Daniel would mean a different kind of dark.

'Please what, Izzy?' Jacob's voice is all game on for some bants, and his eyes are too bright, too lively, too much like what's happening now – and whatever that was, there in his room on his bed – is a game. 'Chill, yeah,' he says, as if I should know that I obviously have no choice but to play. 'Brought you this.' And he's waving what looks like a phone. 'You must have dropped it when we…' So Jacob doesn't know what to call it either. 'Whatever, eh. Sent you some nice *mementos* to keep on here, Fingers. You wanna be careful where you leave it. Prying eyes and all that. You gonna come down?'

'Please.' He's too loud.

'Aw, babe. You want me to come up, is that it?' All those cocksure moves of his are as bold as his volume, which is too much. And I'm telling him no, but he didn't hear it before and he doesn't hear it now because there's a *flick* and a *thud thud thud*, the front door is swinging open and, in the light of the moon, Daniel's up in Jacob's face, hand on his shoulder with a fix that's all *one wrong move, son…*

'Are you OK, Isabel?' Daniel's eyes are on Jacob, his voice level but spiked with that stay-away-from-my-daughter line dads always deliver in those Hollywood movies with those stone-throwing boys.

'Sorry, Mr Chambers,' Jacob says, 'for disturbing you.'

Daniel remains steady, refusing to fill the gaps.

'I was bringing this back for Izzy.'

My heart capsizes, any hope tipping out of it as Jacob shows him the phone.

'Thought this –' he bucks his chin at my window – 'would be quieter than ringing the bell.'

Silence.

'Obviously not though, eh? Sorry.'

'*Just go,*' I want to tell Jacob. '*Please. Just stop talking and go.*'

Daniel removes his hand from Jacob's shoulder, takes my phone, the *mementos*, whatever they are, folded into his palm as he tells Jacob, 'Off you trot then, mate', his Ts like his smile, which is like paper, flat but with those edges that can be painfully sharp.

'You stay where you are, Isabel,' Daniel says.

And Jacob, whose back is to Daniel now, practically glows in the white of the streetlight as he drops his sorry-Mr-Chambers face and quickly presses his tongue in and out of his cheek. 'See you soon, Izzy!'

'Shut that window,' Daniel says to me. 'Now!'

The room shrinks when I close it. And then again when I hear him on the stairs.

I don't take it down, but I touch it, the Jar of Sunshine, fingers slipping from its lid as Daniel comes into my room.

'Jesus, Isabel, it's eleven thirty. Do you not have any consideration for your mother? For me? Here,' he says, a softer tone as he moves to where I'm standing by the wardrobe, his hand on my back a gentle press towards my bed.

Don't make me sit, I think. The give of the mattress always feels too easy when Daniel kisses me goodnight.

'You'd better have this, I suppose.' He holds out my phone.

But I don't want it, not really. Not the *mementos* anyway. I can't let him keep it though, so I reach across and his fingers brush mine and he tells me, 'You need to be careful, Isabel. Remember what I said about saving yourself for someone special.'

When my stepdad's lips press a little too long on my cheek, there's some sick part of me that's relieved Jacob took what he did. That it's done. That it's no longer yet another thing Daniel can take or do. That whatever he does, he's too late for that at least.

Cos that's gone.

EIGHT

The morning sunshine stabbing at the dark of my bedroom is wrong. It doesn't fit with the cold that hit me when I woke. When I remembered.

'Isabel,' Daniel calls, and it's clear from his voice it's a sergeant major's summons, that he's not coming to me, so I go down to the kitchen, where he points at the seat at the breakfast bar next to Mum, saying he wasn't going to do this now, but he doesn't see what choice he has. 'Given the circumstances,' he says.

And I wonder if he knows – if, in the time it took for him to come in from the street and go up to my room, he somehow saw the *mementos* on my phone.

I've deleted them obviously. But they're stuck. In my head. This kaleidoscope of images that just keeps turning and turning, this permanent feed of Jacob and me, Jacob and me, Jacob and me. All on his monument bed. Starting with us sitting on it, his mouth totally 'cheese' while mine is totally straight. *That* picture I could cope with. But the others. It was one thing being there, but seeing it like that, from this different perspective, seeing me there, laid down, eyes closed, legs open – well, it's another opinion, isn't it? A third-party view. And even to me, who was there, who felt it so much I had to stop feeling at all, even to me, in those kaleidoscopic pictures, it looks like I could be game on. There's no battle is what I mean. That Izzy Chambers in the picture? She is flat. Passive. Scum.

Daniel's staring, his chest staying puffed out despite the long exhale of frustration as he makes his way round to the kitchen-counter side of the breakfast bar, his left slipper squeaking with every step. He removes and examines it, takes some superglue from the drawer and squeezes the liquid carefully between the upper and the sole, pinching the two parts together while whistling 'Bring Me Sunshine'. And I swear I loathe him more than ever because that song belongs to me and Grace. She sang it as she filled my jar with the beads of my torn-apart necklace and promised with the lyrics and her heart that there would always be light in the broken pieces, and said that I should never, ever doubt that I was loved.

Daniel whistling our tune feels like theft. Or like he knows somehow that Grace's friendship is as fragile as everything else in my life right now.

'I was going to chat to you about this later,' he says, 'but now seems as good a time as any. What with that boy turning up late last night.' He looks at Mum, like, *you see? You see what your daughter's become?* And the kaleidoscope of images from last night keeps turning as Daniel keeps staring and I keep sinking into this soiled cauldron of hate.

Turning.

Staring.

Sinking.

Turning.

Staring.

Sinking.

The wait is a needle drawing blood, my head whirling like I'm gonna pass out.

'It wasn't even the same boy, was it, Isabel? As the one I saw you with the other day?' He turns to Mum, who's reaching for a second piece of toast when Daniel slaps her hand away. 'What is it with you, Stephanie? You've been eating like a horse. Good job you've got me to keep you in check, eh?' He lifts her hand to his mouth, his lips pressing into the slap mark.

'There's a name for girls like you, Isabel.' His face is a storm, like that one in *The Wizard of Oz* that lifts Dorothy right out of Kansas. Only, Daniel's twister doesn't drop anyone in Oz; it leaves you spinning in the dark, where the familiar sky turns to thin ice and you end up literally shaking.

And I look at Mum, who'll only look at the wall.

He must have seen the pictures. He must somehow know what I've done.

'I got you this,' he says.

And if Mum's been eating like a horse, she now looks as if she's about to bolt like one. Daniel's holding a pregnancy test. The way he holds it makes it look like a weapon.

'Daniel, I —' Mum starts but is cut off by her husband's finger drawing a sharp stop line through the air, which must be too thin for breathing; Mum seems unable to exhale.

'This is nothing to do with you, Stephanie,' he says. 'This is between Isabel and me.'

And out it comes then, all Mum's held-in breath, Daniel too busy sliding the test towards me to notice the release in her.

'I made this point only yesterday, Isabel: do you really want to end up a teenage mother like *her*?' His voice has ratcheted up a notch, like one of those air-raid sirens in the war. 'I got you this as a reminder.' He's so quiet now. So calm. 'Of how terribly things can work out for silly little girls who do silly little things.' He looks from me to Mum. 'Though I thought your own existence would be reminder enough.' He laughs.

It's not like Mum laughs too, but her face? And that sudden easing of her breath? There's relief in it, I'm sure. And I get it, because I've felt the same when Jacob's picked on Grace instead of me. But really? My own mum?

'I'm just trying to help,' he says in that same over-rehearsed voice he uses to run his lines.

'I don't need your help.' I might be saying it to Daniel, but I'm staring at Mum. *I need yours though*, I shout, not aloud, obviously. But there's something in her eyes that tells me she knows. Shit lot of good it does me, but she knows.

'Oh, you need my help all right, Isabel.'

If Daniel knew how little he looks like George Clooney when he's angry, I wonder whether he'd change.

'You both do.' He smiles then, cool and almost disinterested. 'Where would you be without me?' His arms make a cocoon around my mother. 'Same place I'd be without you…' His kisses on her neck so tender, so light. 'Lost,' he says with all that George Clooney charm.

And then he's gone.

'I love you,' Mum mouths. Then, at a volume intended to reach Daniel where he's now climbing the stairs, she says, 'Right, crumpets for breakfast?'

If I thought it would make any difference, I would scream.

NINE

What the actual? Mum's literally making crumpets. I can smell them from my room. Like crumpets are what we need right now. Seriously? Aren't they just going to rile Daniel and make us fat? Make us hate ourselves even more than we do already? And I'd say all that, but I swear there's no point. All I'd get is that wall. The one she makes of whispers. All that *Not right now, Isabel. Later, Isabel. I'm really sorry, Isabel,* but I know that'd be the end of it, cos Daniel would come in and the whispering would turn to silence and any hope of a proper conversation would turn to fear.

So, she's making crumpets and surely she must know that I don't need crumpets right now. I need her.

But you know what? In the absence of Mum I need Grace. You see, the thing with Grace is that she's sound when I'm not. Because when the home stuff gets too much and I feel like I'm gonna lose my shit, she has this way, without even knowing what's caused the explosion, of gathering it back in. She's like a seventeen-year-old-girl-sized version of my Jar of Sunshine, only louder, more decisive and better on the phone.

Today though, she's not picking up, not the first three times I call her at least, and when she does finally answer, it's clear from the elongated, quiet-for-Grace 'Iiiiiiiiiiiiiiiiiiiizzzzzzzzyyyyy' that she's priming me for bad news. 'I *know* we were supposed to be meeting up this morning but…would you *mind*…' she says.

I know that I will but I won't say that obviously, because minding doesn't change things; it just pisses people off.

'I *absolutely promise* to make it up to you.'

Before she even has the chance to break my heart, I break it for her. 'You're spending the day with Nell, aren't you?'

'Not just the *day*, if you agree to cover,' she says. '*Pllllleeeeeeeeaaaasssse.*' And her voice when she asks me to help her have hours in bed with her girlfriend is really no different than it was when she was eight and talking me into lending her my singing and dancing Elmo. 'Nell's parents are away the *entire* weekend and she's planning this amazing dinner with *candles* and one of those *chocolate puddings* they eat on *First Dates* – you know, those *melty* ones that literally look like *sex on a plate*.'

I know this morning's shower will have got rid of them, but I swear I can still feel the greasy crumbs of Monster Munch on my skin. Totally un-amazing. Totally not sex on a plate.

'I've spun Mum this *line* about an English project. You'll *do* it, won't you? Say I'm at *yours*? That we're working on it *together* tonight if she calls?'

When do I ever say anything but yes to Grace?

'Sure.'

'Iz?' And her voice is some kind of metal detector. 'You are *all right*, aren't you?'

I could tell her. About Daniel. Jacob. All of it. Everything I've never mentioned because revelations are like bodies, right? One thing leads to another and before you know it, you're baring all. And I swear it's getting too much, all of this keeping stuff in. Like one more secret and, seriously, I'm gonna go bang.

'The thing is —' I say.

But Grace is all *hold that thought*. And she's really, really sorry, but Nell's on the other line and she's gotta go, but she'll call me back when she can, and I mustn't forget that if her mum phones, she's with me, yeah?

'*Wish me luck!*' she says, even though we both know she doesn't need it.

Will I see you tomorrow? I message her after she's hung up.

And she replies with a thumbs-up and a heart emoji, which is cool, but I know how time tempers things, how all those moments with Mum and Daniel which have been top of my Must Tell Grace pile have slipped into Can't Tell Grace because every normal hour in their aftermath weighs down the idea of talking with this colossal sense of betrayal or shame.

And then there's a fear of Grace disbelieving me too. About Jacob. Cos I walked into his house. I went up to his bedroom. I lay down. Those pictures are proof, right, and I may have deleted them, but he has copies too.

And Daniel? Would Grace believe what I could tell her about him? Because Daniel isn't the kind of man to do these things. Not George-Clooney Daniel who proposed to my mum with a flash-mob dance to Bruno Mars's 'Marry You' in the thrum of Whitstable harbour. I was in on it, carried the roses while *he* carried the ring. 'It was so perfect,' Mum's best mate Becky gushed in the months after, before she stopped being invited over for coffee or wine.

I tried to speak with Becky once, when I saw her in town and she asked how Mum was doing. I tried to explain how Daniel buys all of Mum's clothes and insists on driving her everywhere, but it didn't sound like anything when I put it like that.

'He's always been considerate,' Becky said. 'They're so loved up.' And she looked kind of sad then. 'That's why we see so much less of her these days, I s'pose. She can't bear to be away from him. Don't blame her really.' She winked. 'Why would you want to look at any other face if you had George Clooney at home?'

She smiled, and I smiled and wondered if it wasn't so awful really. Because that was before the worst of it, when I'd still convince myself that maybe it was a misunderstanding, cos Daniel isn't the kind of man who…And Mum would leave him, wouldn't she, if he was?

TEN

You'd think we'd get used to how Daniel shifts, flipping from sunshine to thunder and back again without giving us a chance to look up at the sky. He's all teeth when he comes into my bedroom, no longer the fairy-tale wolf with a pregnancy test but poster-boy Hollywood, whiter than white, holding a pack of cards, asking if I fancy some rummy, or another game perhaps, if I prefer.

'Later maybe,' I say, waving my phone like it's about to ring, which it isn't, obviously, cos Grace is busy, and these days she's literally the only one who ever calls. Her new voice-mail's gone so giggly I felt like I was interrupting a kiss when I tried her just now, so I hung up without saying a word.

Then, miraculously, my phone *does* beep, and Daniel, still with that smile Mum and I both fell in love with, tells me he'll leave me be, and thank god, because the message is from Jacob, only it's not just words he's sent me, but a whole load of flesh too.

Again. Tonight…

It's written in red across a photo of his naked chest, which looks pumped. There may even be oil too.

How do I reply to that? Grace would know. But…

I could ask Hannah and Rosa, only things are still off since one of them screenshotted our conversation about Grace and

Nell, the one where I wondered too loudly if they'd ever remove their tongues from each other's mouths for long enough to do anything other than Snapchat their loved-up faces to the rest of us loveless no-hopes. Luckily Grace hadn't been bothered. 'Cos it's probably true,' she'd said. 'I can't help it – Nell's like *crack*.' And her eyes had dilated at just the thought of her.

I want it. That irresistible urge, I mean. That pull towards someone and the way it lights you up after, how Grace glows as bright as the screen of her phone when a message comes through from Nell. But it's terrifying too, how easily love swallows you and then how easily it can swing the other way.

So with no Grace and no clue, I ignore Jacob and search for some escape in the stranded: in the *Desert Island Discs* Mum listened to on the morning she brought me home from the hospital, sticking on Radio 4 in the hope, she's said in the years since, that those very wise and very adult voices would feed her as she fed me, that their calm would grow her beyond her sixteen years.

I can't imagine Mum that young, a year younger than I am now, shuttled, like some 1950s-shame-on-her-family kind of girl, to the country when her parents discovered she was – how did she say they put it? – Sixteen And With Child. But it wasn't the 1950s – it was the 1990s, very almost the noughties, when Beyoncé was just kicking off with Destiny's Child and Geri Halliwell had already quit the Spice Girls.

She always said the programme's theme tune was enough to take her somewhere that wasn't her grandmother's spare bedroom, somewhere she could stroke my face without someone more adult than her worrying she was being too clumsy or, worse, too motherly, when the hope was she'd still give in to their pleas to hand her baby over to strangers.

'I'd never have given you up,' Mum says, when I ask her to tell me the story for the millionth time in the kitchen later, when I'm fetching the bread and the margarine for lunch, when we're obviously avoiding talking about Daniel's pregnancy-test threat before. 'They couldn't tell me what to do. It was *my* body,' she says. '*My* choice.' And her voice right now is a warning or a weapon – whatever it is, it's something fiercer than I've ever heard from her. And in that there's hope that maybe the defences she built to protect me when I was a baby are still there. But Daniel must've sensed her sudden bolt of backbone too, cos he's like Harry Potter, or Voldemort maybe, apparating from the dining room where he was running through lines to lay a hand on her shoulder and remind her, very gently, of his callback this evening, of his need for quiet, and then, like always, of how he rescued her from that 'bad, bad past'.

He moves back into the other room, not pulling the door to behind him, despite telling us he'd appreciate not being disturbed. So my mum and I, even though I might want to talk to her about Grace or Jacob or, god forbid, Daniel, we basically sit in silence broken only by Grace and her OMG-you-have-to-see-this photo of her and Nell somewhere totally cool, looking totally happy with ten thousand heart emojis and an afterthought that we should totally all go there together sometime.

Totally, I think, and maybe even my face looks sarcastic because Mum breaks the rules of all this quiet and asks if I'm OK.

'Isabel, love?' she says when the only answer I give her is the thump of my phone on the breakfast bar. 'What is it?'

And where do I start, right? Cos the list is endless and it's not as if *she's* not on it. But here I go, knowing better than to voice it so grabbing a pen and paper to write it instead.

Can we go somewhere? To talk?

Before I've even handed it to her, she's shaking her head, like it's not a Post-it I'm holding but a bomb.

'Please.' It's a whisper that's also a beg.

'Not now.' Her fingers have already torn it, my last resort, into tiny shreds. 'Later,' she says, ripping those tiny shreds into even tinier pieces before separating them and shaking them around in the bin.

And I get that she's scared, cos me too. But I've been here before, watching her literally throw away some problem she can't handle.

'You can't get rid of me that easily,' I say. I'm right up in her face so she can't escape the whisper, the hiss. 'I'm not the cat.'

It's clear from how her face breaks that she's remembering how easily she ditched it.

And I'd wait for more *Not now, Isabel. Later, Isabel,* but another message pings in from Jacob.

No skin this time, just: *I shouldn't have to ask twice. Tonight.*

'Isabel?'

I slide my phone into my pocket so Mum can't see it, the threat I thought I'd tempered.

It beeps again.

It's funny how much Jacob wants a piece of me when Mum just threw those dark and broken pieces of me straight into the bin.

ELEVEN

Grace came out when we were, like, seven and she got obsessed with Gabrielle from *Xena: Warrior Princess* after her older sister gorged on the box set twice over one summer holiday, letting Grace sidle in with her on the sofa while their mum and dad either worked or bawled at them to get outside in the sunshine while they still could.

'I don't need *uniform*. I need *leather*,' she screamed at her mother, who was attempting to put an end to our play date so she could take Grace back-to-school shopping in town. 'Xena would *never* love Gabrielle if she were stuck in a blue-and-white *pinafore* and ankle socks.'

'And patent shoes.' *I* was grinning, but Grace's mum, usually so un-stormy, shot me this look like she might go a little warrior herself if we didn't stop with the dramatics.

Even now, Grace pulls the same sulk face as she did back then, her bottom lip pushed out to bare saliva that glistens as it quivers with high-intensity am-dram grief. And god, that pout, it literally pulls the strings on my heart so that whatever she's feeling, I'm feeling too. And my arms have that involuntary reflex thing, like when a doctor bangs on your knee, so I've no choice but to pull her into a hug, not giving a toss about the snot stain she leaves on my top, cos she is Grace

Izzy Ashdown and Grace Izzy Ashdown could never do anything to seriously rock our boat.

Our boat is like the most solid unsinkable boat on the water.

Or it was. These days, the air between us is sort of choppy, and my tummy does that lurchy seasick thing when I lie in bed at night wondering what she's up to with Nell. Because while Grace came out when she was, like, seven, she's never had a girlfriend until now, not a real one anyway, only me dressed up as Gabrielle and I'm no way near as good an actress as Grace and no way near as hot as Gabrielle, so in Grace's eyes at least we were a flop. Romantically, I mean. In every other way, Grace and I have been Academy gold. If there were an Oscar for friendship, we'd have been on that stage shedding our tears and giving our thanks for the last twelve years in a row. Seriously. Even the year she knocked out my two front teeth.

She didn't punch me or anything. Grace doesn't have a violent bone in her body, and believe me, I'd know a violent bone if I saw one. We were running long loops around the playground, chasing girls and boys for kisses, arms in the air like we just didn't care until Grace suddenly did. Care, I mean. Because I was on the brink of catching Emily Lamb, and Emily Lamb, with that cropped blonde hair and those green eyes with a hint of blue – well, Emily Lamb was the closest thing to Gabrielle Grace had ever seen. And while it wasn't like the kisses were proper kisses or that Grace was even thinking the full-on lusty thoughts she thinks now, what it *was*, she says with ten years of hindsight, was her very first prick of gut-blasting jealousy, different to the urge to snatch a toy or whine because her sister had way more custard with her pudding than she did.

She'd only meant to pull me back, not down, and because no one had yet figured out that Grace's eyesight was about as good as a deep-sea fangtooth fish's, she wasn't wearing glasses and didn't notice that I'd made my catch perilously close to the climbing frame and that if I were to fall, which I did, I could whack my face on the slide, which I did, and never see my two front teeth again, which I didn't. And because no one had yet figured out that Reuben Johnson's brain was as dopey as a panda's, no one thought to stop him when he picked up my two front teeth, gave them an actual kiss and tossed them in the conifers so they were gone for good.

'I'm really sorry, Iz,' she said, her fingers assessing the damage as they poked about in my wound. 'I'm such a…' Grace wasn't (and still isn't) often stuck for words. But back then, as my empty-grave gums coloured her nails the perfect shade of danger, she struggled to define her guilt. 'I'm a…I'm…I –'

'Give Izzy some space, please!' Mrs Taylor, of all people, should have known Grace and I never gave each other space. If we could have been stuck at the hip, literally, I swear we'd have slapped on the glue. Grace had even played thick in maths, faked confusion over a pie chart in an attempt to drop down to my set, but our teacher had had none of it because, as we'd once overheard her reminding her colleaguers in the staffroom, Mrs Taylor was 'no goddamn fool'.

'You're my goddamn best friend.' Grace and I would try out Mrs Taylor's American accent and American swears at playtime.

'You're my goddamn hero.'

'You're my goddamn favourite person in the whole goddamn world.'

'I'm goddamn Callisto,' Grace sobbed when Mrs Taylor peeled her away from my gappy mouth and she was under threat of being relegated to bystander like everyone else. Only she was never like everyone else. For a start, everyone else had no idea who or what Callisto was. Grace explained. 'Callisto is the *bloodiest* warlord of all time – she's taken Xena down *over* and *over*. She's so *mean*.' No one but me was any the wiser. And Mrs Taylor, who was goddamn tutting and goddamn shaking her head, had quite clearly had e-goddamn-nough.

But I can't see how anyone could ever have enough of Grace. I mean, look at Nell. She's with my best friend all the time. Literally always hand in hand with her. Thing is, when Nell reaches out for Grace, it never seems needy. Nell's too cool for that maybe. Too sexy too, like so sexy you don't have to be gay to appreciate it. And it's not that she's especially pretty – it's something else. Her smile perhaps, how it comes so easily and so authentically no matter who she's talking to; how her voice isn't dampened by stumbles and sheepishness with someone new. You can tell Nell's listening, and not just listening out for a lull to switch the conversation to her, but really taking it in. It doesn't bother me so much when it's me or one of Grace's other friends she's speaking with, but when Nell and Grace are in deep communion – 'chatting' doesn't do the way *they* talk justice – I choke because it's so obvious, isn't it, how much more Grace has with Nell now than she's ever had with me.

I goddamn miss her. So goddamn much.

My phone, when I pick it up to message Jacob, is like the tarantula I held at some zoo as a kid. All threat and venom, and touching it feels all kinds of wrong.

Tonight then. 9?

I watch the screen for an answer, which doesn't come.

Is that it? Am I off the hook?

I take another shower. Hotter this time. So hot my skin's like one of those umbrellas that changes colour when wet. My chest and my belly turning from chalky mass to scarlet mass in the rush of the water, which, no matter how high I turn the dial on the shower, still can't shift the stickiness of Jacob's hands and mouth and his tongue that slicked those words: 'Relax, Izzy. It'll be so much better if you just fucking relax.' Cos those words, they're as wedged as the earplugs I've used on the worst kinds of nights when Daniel's done what he's done, and he's left, and Mum's crying is as quiet as she can make it, but for all her effort, that sinking weep of hers seeps through the walls like blood on toilet paper.

I leave the water running as I fetch the flannel from the sink, grateful for the steam in the mirror, more grateful even for the barrier the cloth puts between my hands and my flesh, which still stinks of Jacob. Which will stink of him again tonight. Which might always stink of him. Might always feel like him. Like some shitty tattoo. Or the needle that draws it. A million pinpricks every time something – a flannel, body wash, underwear – touches me there.

I daren't put my fingers anywhere close. In the past, Grace has been like: 'Seriously, Iz, *no one's* ever gonna please you if you can't please *yourself* '. And it wasn't like I didn't get it, but Daniel never knocks so it wasn't easy in my room, in my bed, so the shower's been where I've, you know…But this shower, this one right now, is fucking awful, like, really fucking awful, cos it's not getting rid of anything except that one stupid hope I grew here that maybe there was some good in my body, that maybe it wasn't such a big fat dirty waste of space after all.

By the time I'm done and standing naked in front of the mirror, the skin on my chest is as pink as my gums. I have to twist my tongue slightly to slip its tip into the gap between my two front teeth. They came in not long after the Callisto incident, Mrs Taylor using their emergence as a reminder to Grace that me and my body could cope on our own and Grace didn't need to constantly poke her nose (or her finger) into my business. But remembering the photos Jacob has of me on his phone, I'm starting to think Mrs Taylor had no goddamn idea.

TWELVE

It's not like I want 2 spend the night with u, Izzy. Make it 6.

Thing is, I normally run everything by Grace. And I mean everything. But when I call her, just the sound of her hello is a pair of rolling eyes, like, *honestly, Iz, we said tomorrow and you're really phoning me now?*

'My bad,' I tell her. 'I totally forgot you were busy.'

What I really want is for that deep symbiotic connection she swears we live by to kick in so she'll remember to act like my Grace and do the fussing and the organising and the tending I mock but love her for. But, after checking I'm still all right to cover for her tonight while she and Nell go take two on the jiggy in Margate, all she says is 'cool' then she DMs me a blowing-kisses emoji, which I copycat reply with two Xs ('one for you, one for Nell'), because it's better to be kind than to be honest, right?

I should know not to wait right outside the bathroom, where the big bulk of me casts looming shadows across the tiles as soon as Mum opens the door.

'Isabel!' she says, relief saturating her face when she clocks it's only me, and I wonder, nothing new in the thought, if there's pleasure in it for Daniel, in this skill he has of making our hearts snap like twigs with just the idea of him entering a room.

Then he too is on the landing, saying nothing but saying everything, his hand gesturing me first use of the bathroom, his right eye winking as he has enough of my indecision and goes ahead, closing the door behind him, Mum's exhale perfectly timed with the bolt of the lock on the other side.

It's weird, the power of his silence, how calm it can be, and then how fierce. His ability to shift the atmosphere so everyone breathes in his fog. It wasn't always like this. Or maybe it was, maybe Daniel's always atmosphered, only maybe at the beginning the mood he set for us was golden. What I mean is, those first few years are coated in a sort of happy haze, which made a fact of Daniel's love for Mum and me as he placed us at the centre of his universe. Daniel was everything; I heard Mum say as much on the phone to Becky after she came home from a date with him one night, this glow to her face I hadn't seen before, like she'd been showered in glitter and coated in shine.

I'd met Daniel for the first time the following week when he took us to Pizza Express, arriving with a bouquet for Mum and a posy for me, which sounds kind of naff, I guess, but it really wasn't. It was magic, the way he made the two of us walk on air.

'Isabel,' Mum says now, her voice so quiet it's practically Braille, taking me by my hand to my bedroom, like I'm five and she's about to tuck me in.

And I wonder if this is it, if the noise of Daniel's shower is enough cover to let her speak, to tell me something, anything, about that weird shit with the pregnancy test or to ask me about that other weirder shit with Daniel's hands. I'm sure she must have noticed. How the space between us has got narrower. How whatever makes him raise those hands at Mum is making him place them so differently on me. Not as hard, but just as bruising, right?

And I must look at her, like, *ask me and I'll tell you*, cos 'Not now,' she says. Then she whispers, like it's everything, 'Destination moon?'

It's what she'd say when I was little, after George Clooney, the real one, was on *Desert Island Discs*. Mum's excitement about his upcoming appearance must have been catching; I jumped on the sofa with a joy so solid it carved my very first memory upon my brain.

Obviously I didn't realise at the time that, at just nineteen, Mum was young to be on her own in a town with no family but her three-year-old daughter, young to be spending her nights watching American hospital dramas and her weekends listening to *Desert Island Discs*, young to have so much responsibility binding her down. And obviously I didn't realise at the time that, at just nineteen, when she listened to one of George Clooney's choices, Hank Williams's 'I'm So Lonesome I Could Cry', she may well have felt the song was her perfect fit. It would explain the tears, I guess. And maybe what came later, with Daniel too.

I may have been three, but I fell in love with George Clooney that Sunday when we first heard him. Maybe it was his voice, which had a quiet happiness to it, but, really, I think it was what he gave me with his third record: Dinah Washington's 'Destination Moon'. When I listen now, the love in it sounds romantic, but back then, it summed up my relationship with Mum. She made my cares disposable; we could jump in a cardboard-box rocket and leave them far below, because, like space, Mum and her hope seemed endless, and in loving me so fully, she made possibilities seem endless too. After George Clooney Sunday, whenever I panicked about fallen block towers or times tables or some squabble with Grace over which of us could do the best roly-poly, Mum would take me by the hand and suggest we head for 'destination moon'. 'It'll be fine up there,' she'd say, and I'd believe her.

'We can't even see the moon,' I say to her now, pointing at the window, still framing a bright blue and starless sky.

I may as well have slapped her. Sorry but not sorry enough, I open it for the fresh blast of air which stops us both from melting, as the lava of everything we're not saying creeps around our feet, pushing me out of my room, out of the house and on to my phone.

Tick tock, Fingers, says the message from Jacob.

On my way, I reply, the insides of me erupting with earthy volcanic rage.

THIRTEEN

'Sorry? What?' My head's down, eyes to the pavement, avoiding the sky, when Max stops me on the street one away from Jacob's, whatever he was saying blocked by the music in my earphones.

'You're actually doing it then?' Max says for the second time, and he can't be talking about what I think he's talking about, so I just shrug, like, *huh*, and he literally puts into words the thing even Jacob was too polite to name. 'Sleeping with him,' he says, voice like an awkward laugh at some politically incorrect comedian. 'With Jacob!' And he shakes his head then, like Jacob's only gone and pulled this off. 'You know he didn't actually have any photos other than that first Fingers one.' He doesn't even stumble over 'Fingers', like all this is just a normal part of everyone's vocabulary now.

'You what?'

'He conned you, Izzy.' Thing is, Max isn't smug or vicious or mean, he's just, like, *you should have known – we all know what Jacob's like, yeah.*

And I try to say something, but Max's words have torn into my heart and down into my stomach, my head spinning with the kaleidoscope of pictures Jacob would never have had if I hadn't been so stupid. So naive. So me. It must be obvious too, cos Max lays a you-all-right hand on my shoulder, sits me down on a garden wall.

'I can't believe you fell for it. I mean, I know you were pissed at that party, Izzy, but were you honestly that out of it that you couldn't remember what you'd done? Maybe ease up on the drink next time, yeah?'

What else can I say but 'Yeah'?

'You still going? To Jacob's?'

'What choice do I have?'

Max looks at me like it's a given. 'S'pose.'

'He hasn't, you know, shown you anything, has he?'

'Nah, mate. Just told me what he's got. Anyway, least you didn't have to wait until you're twenty-six! Silver linings.'

And I must look at him, like, *you cannot be fucking serious*, cos Max is all 'Sorry, my bad, and I shouldn't make a joke of it, but…'

'You couldn't have a word with him, could you?'

'With Jacob?' And he doesn't have to say anything else cos the snuff of *won't make a blind bit of difference* is clear enough to make his point. 'I'm sorry, Izzy.' And he sounds it too, looks like he'd do something if he could, but this is Jacob we're talking about, right?

'See you later then.' I put my earphones back in but don't bother pressing *play* because, you know what, it feels like all the music has gone.

It's a bit like being at home, cos Jacob and I don't talk, not beyond the 'All right', 'You wanna drink?', ''S OK', 'Come on', 'Won't you just...' and 'Mmmm'. Difference is, here in his bedroom, the quiet isn't burdened with not knowing. We're the opposite of that cos there's no question of what we're here for, of why, less than twenty-four hours after my First Time, I'm back for a second go.

His laptop, rose gold and gleaming, is still open on his desk, streaming films that are different but pretty much the same as before, another heap of those bodies with their compressed wet flesh, mashed into each other like naked commuters on the rush-hour Tube, slick men casually taking from all those blank women unconvincingly up for the game.

Am I up for it? I don't say if I'm not. I lie still, roll when I'm told and drift through Jacob's pleasure, my left hand reaching for the thin strip of light on the floor, wishing the tug of it could pull me up and away to the moon.

It had seemed so reachable when I was a little kid, everything had, before Daniel swept in with his love and his brawn and his gravity.

I let go of the light and give into the weighty cloak of Jacob's body and, you know what, there's a small release in it, in the obviousness and simplicity of what he needs, in how easily he takes it. And even when I see how he's not looking at me but at his laptop, this expression on his face that's not quite pleasure not quite pain, even then it's easy, sort of peaceful, I guess, because the moon isn't an option, because the dark is just that, no glimmer or slither of anything bright.

But then Jacob's grunts go from satisfaction to frustration, and his hands are a desperate grip at my shoulders to keep him going, his face hard, his dick soft, the condom snapped off and into the bin, and his voice slurs my name as he says I haven't done enough, I'm not shaved enough or wet enough, and his eyes flit back to the screen where the guy's monstrous penis stands as raging and red as fire.

It's only then, when the lamp makes light on the barest, ugliest bits of me, that I feel the depth of my hollowness, wondering how I'll ever fill it in.

'I swear it hasn't happened before,' he says, and it's funny, right, how that shame in his voice is the one and only thing we have in common.

I'm pulling my jeans up over my knees when Jacob tosses me my bag.

'Tomorrow, Izzy. Finish what we started, yeah.'

And I nod because, honestly, I think maybe my words are as futile as the music, cos my fate is pretty much done.

FOURTEEN

Despite the still light sky, the moon's kind of huge now, shoving its fullness in my face as I creep out of Jacob's back door, throwing its white light over the big lump of me thudding my way across his garden.

'Head down the side,' he'd said, 'along the fence. No one'll see you there.'

Neither of us mentioned why he seemed so keen on secrecy.

My fingers pull at my phone like it's a magnet, checking for notifications from Grace, which don't come, obviously, cos despite all that bullshit she feeds me about how she'd die – '*literally*,' she says – if we don't speak for, like, an hour, she's found another life source in Nell. Their special night, their 'amazing dinner' and that chocolate fucking pudding are so much more appealing than me.

The ache between my legs is as rough as the ache in my heart because, despite that five-year-old kid in me hoping she might be frantic with me storming out of the house before, there's nothing from Mum.

But maybe she was – frantic, I mean – cos when I turn the corner into our street, she's there, my mum, the same mum who's not really been outside without Daniel in, like, forever. She's right there without him, pulling me into the car, which is parked on the street, only a few seconds' walk from the front door. And she's telling me it doesn't matter that she hasn't driven in three years, because it'll be like riding a bike. And she says this as if it's supposed to be reassuring even though we both know the last time *I* rode a bike, I cut my thigh so deep I needed stitches, and I haven't dared get back on one since. And she says this like the positivity in her words counts for more than the panic in her eyes. And she says this in a voice that's the ratcheting crank of a roller coaster as it nears the top of its highest, scariest climb.

'In the car, Isabel.' And she's not kidding. Her knuckles taut from her hands lugging the bags, already packed for each of us, on to the back seat, she tells me, 'Get a move on – he'll be home soon. It's time to go.'

'OK,' I tell her, 'I'll get in the car.'

And her chest heaves, surging this swell of breath so heavy it makes a rope between us, until I turn to go shut that front door and she shouts at me, 'No!' This too is change, because my mum, the same mum who's not been outside without Daniel in, like, forever, the same mum who talks – if she dares talk – in whispers, says, 'Now.' And her voice is a knife's edge. 'It's time.' Her face, tilted upwards, is cast pale but strong as steel. 'Destination moon,' she says.

And our cardboard rocket is a Vauxhall Astra and our space is the Thanet Way.

FIFTEEN

We're heading north: that's as much as Mum will say for the moment, that and the weird clucking noise she's making with her tongue whenever she has to change gear. And it's not clear if she's pissed off with her driving skills, which are at, like, seventy-eight percent dangerous, or me because I'm twitching with my phone, writing then erasing messages to Grace – nothing to tell her really except Jacob's ruined me and Mum's gone mental, taking me to 'a secret place', like I'm five and she's conning me into a haircut under the guise of a mystery adventure.

'I need to focus, Isabel,' she says and no kidding, right, cos she's already jumped one red light and we're not even out of town. 'Once we're on the motorway, I'll –' She goes quiet then clucks as we approach a roundabout, one hand on the wheel, the other on her chin, nail between her teeth, eyes flicking to the mirror like she's heard sirens. 'I'll explain,' she says but, honestly, I'd rather she concentrate on the road. I'm all for sharing, but I'm all for living too, and we might not be doing either the rate Mum's going: the speed she's driving and the way her knuckles are stretched tight, like we're on an actual roller coaster and she's anticipating the dip.

My phone beeps. She jumps. And I laugh this laugh that's not even funny, cos whatever we have to be scared of, it sure isn't my mobile.

Can we talk?

It's Max. What are we gonna talk about exactly? About his feelings for Grace? My mistakes with Jacob? How it's all my fault for being too drunk and too stupid to stop him?

Jacob's a dick, Izzy.

And yeah, he's totally on to something there, but what of it? Because saying it changes nothing. Not the photos. Not the blackmail. Not the hold Jacob still has over me no matter how far Mum drives. M2. M20. M26. M25. All these roads do is take me further from Jacob and closer, then, to exposure. Because what if Mum keeps on going? What if I can't deliver on my end of the bargain? What if everyone sees those photos? You want to talk about that, Max? Because, you know what, the words mean crap all, and so I've got nothing to say.

'We're not going home.' Mum's voice is a fairground mirror – whatever it's telling me is too wobbly to trust.

'Tonight?'

'Maybe ever.'

And she's got to be joking, right? We can't just up and leave. I've got college. I've got Grace. But worse, I've got that kaleidoscope of photos and a blackmailing dick who'll spread a trail of dirt about me if I don't show.

She reaches over and puts a hand on my knee, but the touch comes a little too late. Those other hands that have been there by now.

Can I call you?

'Isabel, please. Can you just leave your phone alone for one bloody minute.'

71

After everything that's happened, *this* is the thing that makes her angry?

And she must get it, my frustration, because she's softer then, 'It's not safe there.' Mum's voice is pathetic.

No shit, I think, *like, did you seriously only just realise the danger?*

It's clear she wants me to look at her, but I can't cos when I do there are all of these too many words. And I can't say any of them.

'He's only going to get worse.'

Daniel. Jacob. She could mean either of them, talking so slowly, like it's not just me who needs to take in all these things she's suddenly saying.

'I *have* to be there.' My whispers are nothing like my heart, which is pumping. 'I have to be there. My exams,' I say. But what I really want to say is 'Jacob'. My body will be every-where. All spread. Ugly. Seen. And Grace. I'll lose even more of Grace to Nell if I'm gone.

'It's too risky.'

'*Why now though?*' I want to ask. '*Have you spotted it? The way Daniel's hands have been like ivy.*'

We're pulling in for petrol, so she stops the car and shifts to look right at me. 'They've said it'll only get worse.'

'Who?'

'Refuge.'

I must look at her like, *what?*

'It's a charity. For…' She breathes so deep she practically sucks me up through her inhale. 'For domestic violence.'

I hadn't realised the weight of the unspoken until Mum

speaks it, or how the weight of the unspoken isn't just a meta-phor but an actual physical thing, a thing that pulses lighter, if only for a moment, just by saying it aloud.

'I've been calling their helpline.' The ten-pound notes she pulls from her purse shake so hard I can literally hear them. 'They say it's common for the abuse to get much worse when a woman is pregnant.'

'But you're not pregna—' And I think about it, the look on her face when Daniel said that stupid pregnancy test was none of her business. Her relief wasn't that he was picking on *me*, warning *me* not to get pregnant. It was that he didn't know *she* already was.

SIXTEEN

So, this time it's serious: we're going to a refuge. They've given Mum a secret address so Daniel can't track us down. It sounds so movie, so not my life or my mum's, but flashier, like there'll be guns and explosions and girls in tight tops glistening with sweat while men flex their muscles in vests. But while it sounds movie, it doesn't feel it, not in this stuffy car coming off the M25 and on to the M40. There's no glamour in motorways, nor in the reality of Daniel as a hunter, of his fury being so fierce it'd turn my feelings book to flames.

'I don't know,' Mum says, when I ask her what the refuge will be like, whether I'll have my own room, how she feels about having a baby.

'I don't know,' she says, when I ask her when I can next go to college, visit Grace, whether she's booked her first scan.

'I don't know,' she says, when I ask her if she packed my Jar of Sunshine, what Daniel will do when he discovers we've left, how he'll react to being a dad.

'I don't know.'

I wonder if she'd have an answer if I threw myself from the car.

Time was, Mum knew everything. Not only song lyrics but how to use them like medicine, dispensing music to cheer me up, calm me down, make me eat, stop me whining, get me going when I was sluggish or blue. She knew facts too, like what the Little Boy Who Lives Down the Lane was going to do with his bag of wool, how Father Christmas spent the other 364 days of the year and why it takes three days to climb a rainbow. Ask her anything, and she'd have an answer. Plus she was the only mum in my Year Three class who knew how to change the tyre on a car. Seriously, my mum was badass.

'Why don't you play us a *Desert Island*?' she says, either doing the usual and avoiding the subject or proving there's at least one thing she knows and that's a splash of castaway is exactly what I need to mellow, to stop me from asking the bigger question – can I trust you this time? – even though, really, there's no chance I'd ask it aloud. My heart's still cracked from the promises that fell through before.

'Your choice,' she says, and I scroll through the episodes until a castaway's name starts to pull.

The thing about *Desert Island Discs* is its intimacy. Or maybe, more truthfully, the thing about *Desert Island Discs* is that it was a gift from my mum, and so that intimacy isn't only with the guests, it's with the memories of the two of us – when it *was* just the two of us – on those Sunday mornings, when the theme tune would begin and I'd feel happiness in my bones. Literally. It was an actual physical feeling that came with being held, with being trusted to sit quietly, with being able to work out that these people on the radio had struggled, achieved, overcome. There's a light around it, and that light swaddles you when you listen, like the warmth of the island's sunshine, like the truth in the castaways' songs. Cos the other thing about *Desert Island Discs* is the honesty that comes with revealing their tracks, how the guests can't disguise what the music does to them, the way it hammers their body into the shape it was when they first heard it, time-travels them to when they were six or in love or receiving a shot of morphine after accidently setting their halls of residence on fire.

I scroll through the archives, all the way back to the year 2000, when our own story began. And seeing them – the names and the record choices, the dates even – it hits me how these episodes were like the beads of my yellow necklace from Dad. Pre-Daniel, they strung Mum and me together. Mum's parents may have predicted that, as a family of two, she and I would be broken, but by the radio, in the green chair, we were whole.

I pick an episode at random because, really, the guest doesn't matter. What matters is that it's pre-Daniel, and when the *Desert Island* theme tune kicks in, Mum and I are both instantly lulled by 'By the Sleepy Lagoon'. '*I'd pick this,*' I want to tell Mum. '*If I were to compile a playlist of my life, this would be number one. It reminds me of you,*' I want to say to her. I have the words but no strength to explain how it's the sound of happy Sundays at home.

Without the means to say these things aloud, we remain scattered. Silent. Unstrung.

The trouble is, our listening now is spiked with our circumstances: Daniel might not be in the car, but he *is* here, sliding into the castaway's stories and the songs. There's a lyric about a lady looking like a princess, and Daniel's atmosphered from afar. I can feel it, how we both go rigid, remembering how

Daniel said the same of Mum and me, twirling us both by our hands in his kitchen, where he'd laid out this amazing afternoon tea, with cakes and scones and sandwiches with their crusts cut off, something Mum had told him she never did cos she didn't want to indulge my ridiculous demands. I loved it, how he'd even put a tiara on my place mat and a promise on Mum's.

'Oh, Dan,' she'd said. 'I —'

'Daniel.' He'd placed that hand on her shoulder. 'It's Daniel.' And his voice was as sweet as the jam in the Victoria sponge.

'Sorry,' Mum said, 'of course.' She held up the card in which he'd written his promise. 'It's so thoughtful.' Turns out, he'd offered to take me swimming that afternoon so Mum could read, something she'd apparently not had much chance to do since having me. 'My mate leant me the new Caitlin Moran – she says it's —'

'Oh, I got you this.' And Daniel pulled a book from the drawer. '*Jane Eyre*. You're too bright for all that contemporary trash.' He kissed her cheek. 'You want a classic. Of course, if you'd rather read the one your friend gave you…' He went to put the hardback away.

'No, no.' Mum stopped him. 'Give it here – I'd love to read it. The other one can wait. It's so kind of you.'

It was strange to see her hugging someone who wasn't me, but if she was going to hug anyone, I was happy it was Daniel. He made us princesses shine.

'I should have known,' Mum says now, like it would've been so easy not to be fooled by him.

'You can't always tell what someone's like,' I say.

But it's not as if she's only just realised, is it? The clues have been so glaring they stopped being clues and became facts or cuts or bruises.

But I don't say that.

Obviously.

SEVENTEEN

What I do say, when the episode has ended, is: 'What was he like?'

And Mum knows who I'm talking about, because, Daniel aside, there's only been one other 'he' in my life, though 'not in my life' would be more like it.

'He was kind,' she says, not tightening like she normally does if I ask, 'and funny.' She's staring harder through the windscreen now, like it's not the real road she's seeing but memory lane. 'And young. He was the same age you are.' She snaps out of it, looks at my face, and I reckon she's either searching for my real dad in it, or imagining me in the same position as *she* was back then.

I've done it myself, wondered what I'd do, whether I'd see it through like Mum did or go down the route her parents had wanted for her. She's always avoided the A word, as if saying it aloud might make me disappear. Daniel said it once, though, about a year in, not long after my twelfth birthday when he'd whisked us away on the Eurostar to Paris. It'd been freezing but they'd kept each other warm with their held hands and arms wrapped around each other's middles, Mum beckoning at me to keep up cos Daniel had so much planned.

It was on the train journey home. 'Why didn't you have an abortion?' he asked her, and it was kind of weird because we weren't even talking about me – we weren't really talking at all. The focus, for all three of us, was on the game. Daniel had been teaching us rummy and, struggling to get a second run, I'd bought too many extra cards, so my hand was spilling into my lap and to the floor, where Daniel, without even looking down to where I was scrabbling, slid my ace of hearts further away with his foot. Twice.

'Why didn't you have an abortion?' he'd asked.

Even from under the table, I could tell the question was a vacuum, audibly sucking the breath from Mum, who, as I clambered to my seat, shook her head, like, *what?*, but couldn't seem to form actual words for her shock.

'Here, Isabel, you missed one.' Daniel stretched down for the ace and passed it over, kissing my knuckles and winking. 'Let me sort those for you, darling,' he said, taking the mass of cards and arranging the perfect fan. 'There you go: you'll be able to see them all more easily now. Who's for a chocolate button?' he asked and pulled two packets from his pocket. 'For my favourite girls.' He opened one for each of us, occasionally feeding a chocolate to Mum, who'd left hers otherwise untouched on the table.

'Why *didn't* you have an abortion?' I asked her that afternoon as we unpacked the suitcase while Daniel popped out for some milk.

'I couldn't,' she said. 'It was never an option for me, Isabel.'

Because I wasn't as tall as her back then, my ear fell on her chest when she hugged me, her heart thumping like mine when Daniel cajoled me into running on Sundays.

I'm not sure it would *never* be an option for me. If I were pregnant, I mean. I've seen it from the inside, how hard it was for Mum, even before the Daniel thing, how much of the 'normal' she had to give up for herself by not giving up on me. But for me the choice had only ever been theoretical, clearly, cos, despite what they told me in RS, you don't get pregnant if you're a virgin. Which obviously I was until Jacob Mansfield.

I've had sex.

Only 'had' isn't the right word. Not really. Cos it sounds like I've gained something or at the very least like I was actually involved.

And that thought drills through everything else, which is stupid, right, because there's so much other crap happening now, but I can't help it, this thought that if Mum hadn't stayed, or just hadn't stayed so long, if she'd made this decision to up and leave a few days earlier, or if she'd even just told me that this was the plan…If any of those things had been true, then maybe I wouldn't have done the worst thing to my body in some stupid attempt to stop Jacob exposing something he never had. Only now he has it. And the further we drive from Whitstable, the louder '*Tomorrow, Izzy. Finish what we started, yeah*' gets in my head. Louder and louder and louder. Because what Mum doesn't know is, in freeing me from Daniel's trap, she's pushing me further into Jacob's. I won't be there tomorrow. I can't finish what he started.

I'm screwed.

'Isabel,' Mum says, but it's too late. All this leaving and sharing and protecting.

I grab my headphones from my bag, plug them into my

phone and put them in my ears, casting Mum as far away from my island as is possible in this bloody car, looking at her, like, *you haven't learnt, have you? That* patience is not a virtue; it's a risk.

RU OK, Izzy?

Unlike Mum, Max's timing is bang on.

No. You called Jacob a nob but he's so much more.

I know. Can we talk?

Grace isn't interested.

This isn't about Grace.

Well then, I've nothing to say. Leave me alone, Max. You and Jacob and all you lot. Just leave me the hell alone.

EIGHTEEN

Where RU?
   Call me.
   U OK?
   Earth to Izzy…RU hearing me?
   Pick up your phone.
   Seriously, Iz, I need 2 talk 2 u.
   NOW!!!!!!!!!!

It sounds awful, doesn't it, that in the midst of all this, I get this buzz from Grace wanting me, from that ping of her messages as they come through in quick succession when I finally get some reception. And at nine o'clock too. Bang in the middle of her perfect night with Nell. And I *am* tempted to call her, partly to put her mind at rest but mostly just to hear her voice, to get her take on this hurried escape, which has paused with us at another service station, just half an hour from the last, Mum drinking another coffee, one minute saying she's ready but then she's not, drumming her index finger on the handle of the car door like she's all set for making a different kind of run for it.

'Can you just turn that off,' she says when she eyes my phone on my lap.

'But Grace —' I say.

'Not even Grace can know where we're going.'

I start dialling anyway.

'I mean it,' she says.

And I nod, like, *yeah, yeah,* and Mum takes my free hand in hers and squeezes it super hard, like so hard I wince, and her eyes are totally repentant but she doesn't stop, like, *this is it*, until I give her an answer.

'I get it,' I bark at Mum, just as Grace starts in my ear, all high tones swooping into low tones so I can't pick out her emphasis cos it all sounds like a jumble of panic and glee. That's the thing with Grace: she loves a drama. Her mum calls us chalk and cheese. I'm the chalk, I guess; I mean, anyone will tell you that Grace isn't easily wiped away.

'Goddamn it, Izzy. *Where* are you? You *are* still covering for me, yeah?'

And I nod even though she can't see me, and even though I can't possibly cover from however many hundreds of miles away.

'Mum's on her way over to yours. *Now!* She left a message about *ten minutes* ago. I told her about us working on that *stupid* English project and she saw I left my college bag at home. Duh! And now she's *not* picking up her goddamn phone. Must be driving. *Crap.* She must almost be at *yours*, Iz. Just tell her I'm in the *bath* or something, yeah?'

I did promise.

'Izzy? You there?'

There's Nell in the background then, asking if I'll do it, and it's not that her voice is harsh or anything – she just wants to know – but I swear it makes it worse. That *she's* the one check-ing, I mean. That *my* Grace will be shaking her head, like,

Izzy's gone AWOL, and Nell will be totally chill, which will just make my mess look like even more of a shitstorm.

'Izzy! Have you lost your goddamn voice?' And Grace is still kind of joking, but there's an edge to it.

'I can't.' My confession hangs there on the line like a stalactite. Or a stalagmite. Whichever one it is that's just a big old deadly spike pointing down. Like any moment now it might drop and split you in two.

'What do you mean you *can't?*'

I picture Grace, her jaw literally dropped, and Nell, who I can tell is still too close to the phone, still too close to Grace, asking her why I'm not at home now, when I promised I would be. And Nell's voice will be all yoga, just curious in that listening, head-tilted way she has. But Grace. Grace is another story.

'Izzy?'

'I'm sorry.' And I say it maybe three or four times. 'I'm not at home.'

Mum's eyeballing me a warning not to say a word, not releasing that grip, which is starting to feel like a full-on burn.

'Izzy? You *OK?* Are you with *Jacob?* Cos someone told me *something's* going on between you two.' And I can hear it, that break in Grace's rage, the hurt that I've kept a secret, but, more than that, the motherly tone she takes with me when I need her, which is, like, all the time, I know.

'I'm not with Jacob.'

Mum's eyes are practically bleeding with the fix she has on me.

'Izzy?' Grace says, but it's half word, half sigh. '*God*. When did you start *keeping* things from me?'

'I'm not with Jacob,' I repeat. 'Promise.'

'Well, how *quickly* can you get back home then?'

'I'm nowhere close,' I tell Grace, who, with a sharp intake of her breath, sucks in the disbelief and the anger, which get stuck, puffing her up in that way she has of exploding. Nell will have a calming hand on her back, I bet, miming some kind of pranayama exhale, this picture of serenity while smoke practically pours from Grace's ears as she fumes. 'I'm so sorr—'

But before I have the chance to even apologise, let alone explain, Mum – not risking any more, I guess – snatches the phone from me and puts an end to the call.

'If she phones back —'

Before Mum can finish, it's already ringing again. She holds it away from me, tucks it down between her seat and the door.

'You can't tell Grace anything.' And I'm nodding, but she goes on anyway. 'I've never been more serious, Izzy.'

She hasn't called me Izzy for years. I don't know when exactly I became permanently Isabel, but it was sometime after Daniel arrived, when he said how beautiful our names were. Wasn't it a shame, he said, that people couldn't be bothered to say them in full? Would we mind, he asked, if he made us Stephanie and Isabel? Because the last thing he wanted was to cut the two of us in half.

Mum's friends persisted with 'Steph', but only while they were still on the scene, which became less and less often as

Daniel found reasonable excuse after reasonable excuse why dinner with Claire couldn't work that night, why the cinema with Becky just wouldn't do. Sociable Steph gradually became unsociable Stephanie until Claire and Becky had dropped away and Steph was lost, cast on a desert island shaped like another time.

'OK,' I say to Mum, and that look on her face! Like it's not my phone she's putting in my hands but her life.

'Grace.' I take the call and the fire that comes with it.

'You *promised* me, Iz. Seriously, everything I do for *you* and you can't do this! Are you *sure* you're not with Jacob? Cos if you've let me down for that *prick*, I *swear...*'

'I'm not with Jacob,' I repeat, comforted by the truth of it.

'So where are you?'

'I can't tell you. I'm sor—'

'*Can't* or *won't?*' And her voice is a mind made up. 'You know what *I* reckon? I reckon you're so *jealous* of my relationship with Nell that you've done this on *purpose.*'

'That's not true. I promise, I —'

'So you're *not* jealous then?'

'No.'

'*Liar,*' she says. 'I can hear it in that *pathetic* little voice of yours. You can't hide *anything*, Izzy.'

And if only she knew, right? Cos Grace thinks she's got this sixth sense or whatever, but what kind of friend is she when... yeah, I may not have said anything out loud, but what about all those other ways I've tried to let her know I need her? Like when Jacob Mansfield had me pinned to a radiator with his hands in my knickers and all she said was sorry. Not even to me but to him. For interrupting. What about that?

'You know what, Grace? I *didn't* do this on purpose. But I'm glad you're getting caught. Serves you right.'

And she's not the only one with gut feeling cos I'm pretty sure her hanging up means she's sending me to goddamn hell.

'What's happened?' Mum's hands are cold when she tries to shake out an answer from me.

The cover of that feelings book flickers in my mind, the same little girl repeated to make a circle of little girls, her different moods drawn on her otherwise identical faces. One second I'm the one with downturned lips and tears, the next I'm all clenched fists and a mouth so wide and so fierce I'm breathing fire.

'I let her down,' I spit the flames, 'and I've no chance of making any of it better because of this.' I point at the suitcases on the back seat. 'Because of *you*!' And my stare's as hard as a slap, I reckon, cos Mum recoils the same way she does when Daniel snaps.

And despite the shame of it – of being like him, I mean – I'd go on. Honestly, I would. But Mum bites her lip, starts the engine and rejoins the motorway, taking me further and further away.

NINETEEN

When I close my eyes, I'm the furthest away from everything. Mum included.

This blind darkness with flashes of headlights. Just me. On my own.

Time was, I was never alone; Mum or Grace were always beside me, like stabilisers. And I know stabilisers are only supposed to be temporary, that they're meant to come away when you're ready to ride independently, but I'd never expected them to disappear completely, had assumed they'd remain either side of me, each propping me up when I was at risk of a fall.

I can't remember the specific moment I lost the first one, maybe because as Mum gradually became less able to prop me up, Grace stepped in and supported me from both sides: as Mum went out less, Grace came over more; and as Mum's voice grew softer, Grace filled my own quiet with her non-stop talking. Not that we ever talked about *that* because there wasn't really much I could say, nothing in particular I could point out that was hurting Mum. Cos it's not like there were bruises, not then.

And I hadn't even noticed what Grace was doing. That she was being a double prop, I mean. It was only when her mum said something last year, when we were taking our GCSEs and Grace was calling me each morning to remind me what exam I had that day, meeting me at the school gates to check I had the right stationery and waiting afterwards to reassure me I'd done OK.

'You'll make an excellent mother one day, Grace,' her mum, Marion, had said when we were done with exams, eating jam-drippy scones and filling in the online form for our celebratory change of name. 'Izzy, how on earth will you get yourself through a degree if you and Grace opt for different unis?'

And we'd just laughed, cos like that was ever gonna happen.

'You know, I think Grace has been a better parent to you, Izzy, than I've been to her the last few years!'

I'm not even sure Marion was joking. She was smiling though, shaking her head as she pulled up a chair next to us, twisting Grace's laptop round so she could take a proper look. 'Are you girls really going through with this?'

'Yep!' we said in perfect unison.

'We've been practising our new signatures!' Grace slid the A4 sheets scrawled with *Grace Izzy Ashdown* and *Izzy Grace Chambers* across to her mum. 'Cool, right?'

Marion and Grace didn't pick up on the legal change of Isabel to Izzy too. And I mentioned none of it to Mum, cos it's not like she was ever gonna remember the promise Grace and I made when we were, like, ten, that we'd give each other our names, proof that we're as good as family. Better even. So Grace is me and I am Grace. She is my rock with my name running right through her middle.

But rock's not totally indestructible, right?

If the fall of my first stabiliser went almost unnoticed, the second? Well, its retreat was much more of a bang. 4:37P.M. on 13 February 2017, the minute Grace first swiped right on Nell. '*Take note of the time, Izzy*,' she called down the phone. '*I've just clocked the love of my life.*' I should've known it was trouble when not just the odd word but her whole sentences were inflected.

It's not like she just disappeared, and Grace probably doesn't even realise anything's changed, but *something* has definitely changed, and not because of tonight's phone call. Before then. Because a few months back I'd have had no hesitation in telling her what happened with Jacob and, by this stage, maybe I'd have even told her what's happening with Mum. But for some reason now I'm freewheeling.

I wonder how different it would be if I'd really known my dad, if he'd been someone I could call when Mum and Grace's lines were otherwise engaged, whether he'd have offered me a home when Daniel's turned into a prison, whether he'd have been happy that it was never an option for Mum or if he'd ever have asked the same question as Daniel in the hope that saying the A word aloud might just make me disappear.

When the *Desert Island* episode ends and 'By the Sleepy Lagoon' swoops in once more, I close my eyes and imagine myself on the island, drifting away from everyone and everything I know.

When I open them again, it occurs to me that I don't have to close my eyes and imagine. Because with this car, this journey, this mystery destination, Mum's already created an exile of her own.

TWENTY

If things had been different, maybe I could have told Mum, *'Screw you and your too-late worry.'* *'See you in a day or so,'* I'd have said, when things had calmed down. *'I'm off to Dad's now,'* I'd have told her, and headed south to Brighton instead of north to Location X.

And if things had been different, maybe my dad would've opened his door and his arms, and my half-brothers and -sisters would've come running to see me, pulling at my legs and my hands, wanting to show me their Lego sheep or a fairy they'd made from leaves, or the headstand they'd been mastering since they saw me that last time at the woods when, if things had been different, maybe we'd have enjoyed the tastiest picnic in the warmest sunshine and chased butterflies and played hide-and-seek in the trees. If things had been different, maybe Mum could have been there too, and the half-brothers and -sisters could be whole, and other picnickers could have commented on our red hair and our pale skin and said weren't we a picture, how we all looked so much like our mother but sang just like our dad. Because if things had been different, maybe he could have brought his guitar and let us all take a turn and we'd play our top tracks or sing a family favourite not quite in harmony, but it'd feel like magic with our voices so together, so aloud.

Things aren't different though. Things are what they are, and I can't go to my dad's because my dad…well, my dad is dead. Yeah. Sucks, right? And you'd think I couldn't grieve for someone I didn't know, but I do, always, because if that one thing – his death – had been different, I'm fairly sure pretty much everything else would be too.

Mum was ready to move on. From me being a dirty secret, I mean. Because by the time I was, like, four or five, she was strong. She had this job in the bank and these friends who popped by with dinners in tubs for the two of us, using words like 'tough' and 'cope' and 'Honestly, Steph, I've no idea how you do it alone'. They admired her, they said, how she was always so happy, and Mum would cock her head at me and say, 'How could I not be?', and her friends would smile and nod and arrange to meet up for coffee or wine, and they'd come back over with a bottle of white and a barrel of questions, and I'd listen through the thin walls of our flat as Mum chatted to them so freely about stuff she avoided with me.

And all that talk, it led her somewhere new, somewhere things *could* be different, somewhere things might not be so tough, somewhere she could do more than just cope, somewhere she might not have to do it alone. And so she sat me down with a Bourbon biscuit and told me she'd found my dad.

'He wants to meet you,' she said, and hope suddenly tasted like the brown crumbs I was picking from my knees.

We met just the once, when I was five, and he was everything she'd said he would be: tall and smiley and smelling of an aftershave Mum later told me was L'eau D'Issey Pour Homme.

The three of us went to the park, and I remember being high on the swing looking around at all the other kids, expecting them to be looking back at me, at this man who was my actual real-life dad standing right there behind me, pushing me closer and closer to the sky. And I thought their jaws would be dropping at this miracle. But no one else could see it. And I guess that's when I first realised how small our lives are, how no one really sees anything but the obvious, how people rarely look beyond their horizon or ask questions of others in an effort to reveal their truth.

But my dad did. Ask questions, I mean. And not the usual 'How do you like school?', 'What's your favourite TV show?' and 'What's the name of the teddy you're holding there?' Instead he asked me: 'When are you the closest to physically bursting with glee?', 'Do you think you're a good friend?' and 'Do you like music and why?'

That last question was the key that unlocked my voice.

'Yes,' I said. 'My favourite song is by Dinah Washington. George Clooney gave her to me. And she takes me and Mummy to the moon.'

'Maybe I could come next time too?' he said.

I looked at Mum because I was crap at making decisions even then.

She nodded.

'I could give you a song as well if you like,' my dad said.

For once I didn't need guidance. 'Yes, please,' I said.

And my dad, my dad who didn't know I existed until one

week previous, my dad who'd driven all the way from Brighton with an almost-empty photo album and a battered but tuned guitar, my dad, my actual real-life dad, sat down on our living-room floor and sang 'You Are My Sunshine', and I felt the light of his actual real-life love.

He died one week later when he was on his way to see me a second time. In the boot of his car were three strings of yellow beads and a copy of Carly Simon's *Into White* album all wrapped up and labelled with my name.

Dear Izzy, The colour of these necklaces reminded me of you. Keep the sunshine close to your heart. And track number eight – it's all true. With lots of love, Daddy.

I only cried that day because Mum did. Because why would I cry for a man I'd met only once? But when Mum bought us a record player just so I could listen, I got it: the music hit me with what I'd lost. We played 'You Are My Sunshine' on my birthday, his birthday and the anniversary of his death. When the record player got damaged not long after we'd moved into Daniel's, I searched for the song online and found all these other versions, and while Carly Simon's will always be special, it was never quite right because she just couldn't get close to sounding like my dad sitting on our living-room floor making me believe I was as great and as bright as the sun.

As I got older, I played various covers on my way to school, on my way home from school and whenever the moon Mum and I were destined for was hidden from view. Johnny Cash was too gruff; the Soggy Bottom Boys were too old. And then one day, when the sky was grey as lead, Grace sent me this version she found by these two guys Dan and Charlie on

YouTube who nailed it like my dad with a ukulele and guitar. If I close my eyes, I can just about believe it's him singing, and though my skin is totally goosebumped, I'm warm.

What's best about Dan and Charlie is they only sing the nice bit, the same bit my dad sang to me. Those other verses, about disappeared sunshine and shattered dreams, they're too much like reality, too close to the bone.

So it's only that light-filled part of the track that belongs to me. And I *do* reckon a song *can* belong to a person as much as a necklace or a cat or a book, more so even, because a necklace gets broken, a cat gets given away, a book gets ripped apart. I guess that's why you'd want music on an island, because music is immortal whereas people aren't. Because even when you don't have the record player or even the record, you have your voice, which was unlocked by your dad, who met you just once when he made you the light in his sky. And you can sing.

But yeah, if things had been different, I'd have had more than that song, more than the photo album in which my dad put a picture of him and Mum when they were seventeen and sixteen, along with a note telling me how the idea of filling the pages with photos of the two of us put him the closest he'd ever been to physically bursting with glee. If things had been different, Mum's heart wouldn't have broken with losing him a second time and the hole he left wouldn't have been filled by a man who shines like sunshine but flattens like a typhoon.

If things had been different, Daniel wouldn't have pulled so hard at the necklaces that the strings snapped and the beads scattered across the floor.

If things had been different, Mum and Grace would still be my stabilisers, we'd still be strung together, and I'd be more than all my broken pieces, wearing the sunshine close to my heart rather than storing it in a jar.

If things had been different, an imaginary island with music would be refuge enough.

But they're not. It's not. We need an actual real-life refuge because things are what they are. The photo album is empty. The sun doesn't shine. We can't sing.

Maybe I should have stuck with the Carly Simon version of 'You Are My Sunshine' that Dad gave me, not tried to kid myself that I was due anything more than heartache. danandcharlie95 may have gleaned the happy bits, but life's not like YouTube, is it? Life is how Carly and Johnny sang it: the sunshine goes when the people you love find some-one new.

TWENTY-ONE

We arrive on a dark suburban street where some woman, whose hand is on my shoulder as she tells me her name's Elizabeth, takes us from our car into a house which feels nothing like home. Whatever home is. And I know she's doing her best to make us welcome, with that smile she has, which is just about perfect in that not-too-jolly-but-totally-warm kind of way that I guess this situation calls for.

This situation!

It sounds so dramatic, right? We have a situation! Like the police are about to swoop in and put up a do-not-cross cordon before taking evidence and ushering us into witness protection. But, no shit, we're not far off. Because Elizabeth's giving us some 'basic rules', and Mum wasn't kidding when she said about not telling a soul where we are.

'For your own safety,' Elizabeth says, 'and for the safety of the other women and children here, we ask that you don't give anyone your address. We'd also appreciate you turning off the location services on your mobile, if you have one.'

Mum looks at me, like, *hand it over*, but my hand stays wrapped around my phone, willing the vibration of a message from Grace. Nothing comes, not during Elizabeth's speech or when we dump our stuff in 'our room', or when she's looking at her watch, asking do we want tea cos it's almost midnight, and maybe we'd rather go to bed and run through everything in the morning.

But Mum's too wired, she says, her eyes wide and her mouth kind of open, like there's so much story waiting to spill. So Elizabeth boils the kettle, running through the list of services available to us while we're here. There's a whole heap of people we can meet on Monday apparently. 'They're all here to help,' she says. And though I like her, I want to shove the packet of Rich Tea Elizabeth's offering me in her face, because it's not that simple, is it? It's not just one thing. It's Daniel. It's Jacob. It's Grace. It's too many goddamn beads scattered in different directions across the floor.

We're too far away for starters.

All those miles we've driven, they burn in my heart like that entire jar of silver-skinned pickled onions Grace and I shared between us two summers ago, seeing how many we could squish into our mouths at once, dribbling thin lines down our chins as our vinegared giggles brought Daniel up to my room, where he told Grace, 'Even with the drool, you're just like a young Nathalie Emmanuel.'

'Aw, thanks,' she said, one hand self-consciously toying with her 'fro, all uncharacteristically coy, because after Grace's crush on Gabrielle came her crush on Missandei. '*Game of Thrones!* I didn't know you were a Thronie, D!'

He didn't correct her either – none of his usual 'It's Daniel'. Just a wink and 'I like to be a man of mystery, G.'

D?

G?

I remember how the acid on my tongue spread to my chest. Fast. Vicious. Raw.

'He's *so* goddamn cool,' Grace said after she and Daniel spent twenty or so minutes narrowing down their favourite *Game of Thrones* episodes to 'The Dance of Dragons' or 'Baelor'.

'As a goddamn iceberg,' I said, thinking of that unexposed mass lurking beneath the water. I was so close to telling her. 'You know, ninety percent of an iceberg is underwater,' I said.

But Grace was back on her phone. 'OMG, Izzy! It's not all about *scissoring*!! In fact, this suggests it's almost *never* about scissoring!'

'Huh?'

'Sex! Girl sex, I mean.'

'Grace, are you on Autostraddle again?'

And she was, obviously, because ever since she'd discovered it, Grace had been banging on about this 'kick-ass lesbian and bi site' where she was learning everything she needed to know about being 'the best *bloody* queer I can be'.

That's the thing with Grace: whatever she does/is, she does/is it with gusto. That's why I'm so vexed about her sending me to goddamn hell: Grace never promises something and doesn't see it through.

'Make yourselves at home,' Elizabeth is saying for the third or fourth time, 'but do think of the other women and kids here and tidy up after yourselves, please. It's important we all work together to keep this place nice.' She's leading by example, washing our cups, putting the biscuits in a tin. 'Oh, Kate, hi,' she says, as the slick stick of bare feet on lino comes into the room behind me.

'All right.' The woman might be twenty, she might be forty; it's hard to tell cos her face is so puffy, so bruised. Her left eye is barely open, and the cheek below sags like it's been dragged off its bone, pulling at the corner of her mouth in a way that reminds me of Grace's nan after her stroke, but more savage. 'I'm Kate,' she says, lisping a little, and I try not to stare at the chipped front tooth when I take the hand she offers, try not to wince as she moves closer and the red around the iris of her right eye mottles with the white so it looks like that lining at the bottom of a packet of fresh steak. 'It's OK,' she says, and her other teeth are so straight, so perfect, it's like they couldn't possibly be part of the same face, 'you can look. A bit Frankenstein, aren't I?'

'Frankenstein's monster actually,' Mum says, and I must look at her like, *that's a bit rude*, cos she's all sorries and *I don't know what I was thinking*s. 'I'm Stephanie by the way…Steph actually.' And when they shake each other's hands, Mum's face is like one of those kids at school waiting to be picked for the team. 'Frankenstein's the bloke who created the monster, not the monster itself.'

And I'm seriously like, *just stop it!*

But Mum offers Kate, who sits down next to her, a biscuit, and the two of them turn their chairs a fraction so they're more easily able to talk.

'So I'm the monster then?' Kate's laughing though and her voice is all genuine curiosity, like Grace on Autostraddle getting wise to something new.

'Oh god, I didn't mean it like that. I'm sorry.' Mum's head is in her palms in total embarrassment.

Kate reaches over, takes one of Mum's hands, and they look right at each other, like there's some kind of understanding. 'He might be Frankenstein but, to be fair, he's a bit of a monster too.' Kate winces slightly as she chews on the Rich Tea. 'Though I can think of a few other names I'd call him if I saw him.'

'I know what you mean.'

Maybe I've gone total loco here but are we actually sitting around a table with smiley Elizabeth and bruised Kate making jokey small talk about what to name the men who've ruined our lives?

'Elizabeth's right: it's late.' Mum looks from her watch to me. 'I should get you to bed, Izzy.'

This is a joke, right? I'm seventeen. Mum hasn't put me to bed for years, hasn't even come in to say goodnight since Daniel insisted on her ten o'clock lights out. Seriously! And what? She goes back to 'Izzy' and all those years are undone? She starts acting like mother of the year, when there are so many other things she should have concerned herself with before my bloody bedtime.

'Nice to meet you, Izzy.'

'Night,' I say to the floor, cos, not being rude or anything, but I can no longer look at Kate's face when she talks to me.

Daniel was careful, you see – he kept Mum's 'accidents', as he sometimes called them, to places where they could be hidden under clothes. Made them easier to ignore, I guess, whereas Kate – well, her hurt's totally exposed.

'You stay here if you like, Mum.' I don't mean for it to sound quite so much like that's what I want.

'No, no,' she says, all awkward now, like I've revealed something just as painful as cuts and bruises. 'We both need some rest.'

And none of it feels true. Not the way she reaches for my hand as we leave the kitchen. Not the whisper that the room is quite nice really, isn't it. Not the way she says 'Izzy', which sounds as thin and as forced as her promise that 'Honestly, Izzy, I mean it this time. I promise you, Izzy. We'll be OK.'

TWENTY-TWO

We've been here before. Not here exactly. Not a refuge with an Elizabeth, a Kate and Rich Tea biscuits, but a hotel room littered with a few of our belongings and all of our hopes that things would be different from now on. I swear that's what Mum said that time three Christmases ago when she whisked me away like she did tonight and took me to a Premier Inn. 'Things will be different from now on,' she said, and I believed her. Back then I had no reason not to.

But it didn't take long for Daniel to find us, knocking on the door, his taps so much softer than you'd imagine, and even the way he said Mum's name was a plea. 'Steph,' he said. 'I need you.'

And the door must have been made of aspirin or something, cos the memory of all that pain he'd caused seemed to dissolve with his noisy tears so that he was in the room then, on his knees, literally begging cos he couldn't bear to be without us, especially now, he said. 'My mother's died.' And not being harsh but that news was a done deal, right? 'Very early this morning.' He was weeping. 'In her sleep.' Properly weeping. 'At least it was peaceful.' Like full-on, couldn't-catch-his-breath kind of weeping. 'I need you.' And so it didn't matter that Mum hadn't yet let herself look at him, cos his howls were like the barks of a sheepdog or something, calling her, drawing her in. 'I can't be without you. Not now.'

I went to sit in the bathroom like Mum told me, but the walls were as thin as my hopes were by then.

Only she could save him, he told her. And so we put our things back into the suitcases and Mum let me take the tiny shampoo and the tiny shower gel from the tiny bathroom, maybe as tiny compensation for not seeing through that tiny hope she'd given me. 'It will be better,' she whispered.

It wasn't just miniature toiletries I took from that hotel. I took a lesson too: Mum couldn't be trusted. Not in the slimy way you don't trust a liar or the sceptical way you don't trust a drunk. She wasn't conniving, deceitful or mean.

She was hopeful, I guess, and I got it, cos Daniel's not one hundred percent nasty – he lights scented candles, makes dinner, whisks us away to Paris, brought us into his home and says sorry. 'He's a romantic,' Mum said once. 'He feels things deeply.' '*No shit*,' I wanted to shout. '*So do we*.' But he cries too. Big heaving lumps of apology spill from his chest when he's done what he's done and you believe him, because he's broken, he says. Can we help fix him? he asks, and monsters, real monsters, they don't want your help or your forgiveness, not like Daniel who wants it all, needs it all if he's to have a chance of getting better, of becoming the kind of man we deserve.

Before Daniel found us, when we hadn't been in the hotel room long, we were lying on the bed listening to a *Desert Island Discs* when Mum said, 'Destination moon', and even though I was almost fifteen, I snuggled into the curve of her spoon-shaped body and let the warmth and the smell of her take me to that place I hadn't let myself sink into for years, that sweet spot where Mum put *me* first. And it's weird, cos I hadn't really realised I wasn't there – in that number one spot, I mean – until we left the house early that morning. And when Mum ushered me, an hour later, from the car into the hotel, neck like an owl as she looked for signs of Daniel, and whispered, 'I'll keep you safe', I hadn't thought that she hadn't been. Keeping me safe, that is. I hadn't put any of the responsibility for my unhappiness with her. It was all down to Daniel, right?

It's like riding a bike, I guess, that ability to feel safe again: all you need is the vehicle and your body remembers the rest. The muscles relax, the heart slows and the trust, in your mum and in yourself too, unravels from that tight knot in your stomach and unwinds its way, like cotton, to your Mum's hands, which hold just enough of your weight that you let yourself believe you won't fall.

Like I say, everything went back in the suitcases that went back to Daniel's, but that trust? I'm not sure where it is any more.

TWENTY-THREE

'Did Daniel ever hurt you, Izzy?' Mum's voice from where she lies on the bottom bunk is like her fingers on my neck when she's searched for sore and swollen glands. All those tender tentative prods.

I think of that woman earlier, how her face was like a map of someone's cruelty. 'Not like Kate.'

'There are different kinds of hurt.'

I'm not sure I'd known what it was before, that fear that became like smoke, how it was almost invisible when it started, all soft and wispy, and you could pass it off as something else because the fire was masquerading as something different too.

'He never hit me.' And that's true. Daniel did all sorts of things to my mum, but the hands he laid on me were another kind of intrusion.

'Was there anything else though? Because sometimes…I don't know. I just wondered if he ever…'

What do I say to that? She knows how Daniel works. How the things he did before he kicked or punched her were way too subtle to explain. How they could so easily be a misunderstanding. How his eyes on my chest were because I'd stained my top with toothpaste. And he was only helping, wasn't he, when he licked his fingers and tried to rub it clean.

How his hands on my shoulders were a stress-relieving massage and his mouth on my ear was Chinese whispers. A game.

'I had to get you out,' she says, like maybe this flight for destination moon is about more than Daniel and Mum. Maybe it's also about Daniel and me.

'It was…' But I don't know how to tell her that it felt like he was laying foundations, building up to something so awful it might black out the sky.

'But he never —' she presses.

'He didn't actually —'

'OK.' But it doesn't sound it. Like she thinks this is OK, I mean.

I put all our unfinished sentences in the chest of drawers with the stuff I unpack from my bag.

'It's almost one, Izzy,' she says. 'We can sort all of this in the morning.'

'Where did you put my sunshine?'

I hadn't noticed Mum had drifted off until she startles with the question.

'Mmmm, what?' And there it is, that fraction of a second when she isn't sure where she is, or how dangerous the thing that made her jump might be.

'My sunshine, Mum. I can't see it.'

She's sitting up, but there's no urgency to her movements, this expression on her face like, *look at the mess you're making*, but doesn't she get it? That there's a reason I'm pulling everything from the bags? That I'm looking for a glimmer of light?

'I need it.' And I say it like she knows how every night I take one bead from the jar and put it beneath my pillow.

'Oh god, Iz, I'm so sorry,' she says, shifting to stand.

I say, 'It's fine', even though we both know it isn't.

I want it to be true. That it's fine, I mean. Because in the grand scheme of things, it's just a jar of beads, right? But some things aren't just the things they seem to be: they're the feel of something that was, and the promise of something that could have been too.

I'd worn those yellow string necklaces my dad had for me in the boot of his doomed car almost every day for nearly nine years. Even when uniform ruled them out during school hours, they became part of my bedtime routine, clattering against my chest beneath my pyjamas, my fingers counting the bumps of them as Mum read me *Harry Potter* until my eyelids began to droop and she'd close the book then lift them over my head, careful, careful because their sunshine was even more delicate in the dark. When the bedtime stories stopped, I wore them just the same, ignoring Mum's warnings and falling asleep in them sometimes, because if I pretended hard enough the indentations they made on my skin burnt a direct path of sunshine to my heart.

Daniel said it was an accident. Of course he did. Just like he said sorry too, not just once but maybe five or six times, as he chased the hundreds of yellow balls across the floor. Mum said we'd find another one, and we probably could have done, cos they weren't special, just cheap plastic and gaudy yellow, the kind of thing you'd pick up in a pound shop. But the point was, my dad's hands had held them. It wasn't only those beads that were connected by the string.

I knew not to cry by then, that tears were like rubbing salt in the wound of Daniel's temper. 'It's OK,' I said and wrapped them in tinfoil, repeating how it was an accident when Grace appeared singing 'Bring Me Sunshine' and bearing a jam jar with a screw-tight lid.

The Jar of Sunshine sat on my shelf between a stack of Mum's old Judy Blume novels and a photo of Grace holding my cat Sinitta like it was a baby.

'That thing looks so morbid,' Daniel said, when he came in to check I was working to the revision timetable he drew up for me last year, 'like an urn.'

I hid the jar inside the wardrobe then, not because it *was* morbid but because nothing seemed safe any more.

I wonder if Daniel's found it. If he searched for Mum and me when he realised we'd gone, trawling for clues through cupboards and drawers, pulling at their contents as hard as he's pulled at Mum's hair sometimes, mindful not to catch his nails on her skin.

I know there are worse things in the world than leaving a jar of beads.

But.

'Are you stupid or what?' And it might be a mutter, but the room is a box.

'There was barely any time,' Mum says, and what I hate most is it's the voice she uses when Daniel's on the brink, when she and I will both go over-the-top calm so as not to stir anything else in him.

'But the jar, Mum. It's…It's…' I can't say what it is. What it means. And all those inadequate words mash into some kind of growl so hard it hurts my throat, before I quickly pull it back in again, not wanting to spit my emotions on the floor.

It's something like shame, the way she won't look up from her nails as she picks at the surrounding skin. She used to wear this bright varnish. 'Happy hands,' she'd say, waving her freshly painted fingertips like finger puppets, until one December afternoon, after he'd lit the wood burner and dished up his home-made carrot and coriander soup, Daniel pointed at a photo of some celeb in *Heat* and scoffed at their 'trashy neon nails', said how he'd stick them straight in the magazine's circle of shame. He didn't mention Mum, or look at her even, but those blues, yellows and pinks of hers – well, they were gone.

None of these things seemed to matter much at the time, but looking back, I reckon comments like those were Daniel's own red pencil, each scratching a tiny part of the circle of shame he was drawing around my mum.

'I'm sorry, Iz,' she says, sliding under the duvet even though she's still in her jeans and that tartan shirt I haven't seen her wear since, like, forever. 'I only had an hour to get our stuff together so we could leave. I couldn't do it when Daniel was there.' That red circle Daniel drew around her is like barbed wire sometimes; it cuts just to think of her climbing out. 'You know how tricky he makes things.'

How *tricky* he makes things? *Tricky?*

'*Algebra's tricky*,' I feel like shouting, but she's closing her eyes again so, obviously, like always, right, I say nothing at all.

TWENTY-FOUR

Although the pillow's not my pillow and the bed's not my bed, it's easier to lie in this room in this refuge in this dark. I don't say this to Mum, maybe because she might already be sleeping, but maybe cos there's this streak of me that doesn't want to tell her she's done some good. Because maybe she has – done some good, I mean – but she could have done it sooner. Before the lying down and taking it from Jacob. Before the deal was struck. Before the fingers photo. Before the party. Before Daniel even started on the eyes and the hands on me. Before he even thought of coming to my room most nights, sitting on the edge of my bed and telling me how much he loved me. How I was the reason he stayed, how it wasn't Mum he was here for, cos hadn't I noticed how strange she'd become, how isolated and angry? 'Aren't we lucky, Isabel, that we have each other, that through all this luck and coincidence, you became my girl?' 'My girl,' he'd say, over and over, 'my girl', stroking my face and my hair and my shoulder, as I edged down beneath the duvet, imagining the Jar of Sunshine in my wardrobe and counting the yellow beads. Two hundred and twenty-eight minus the one beneath my pillow, which I'd roll between my fingers as soon as he left the room.

And all that 'my girl, my girl' could be sweet, right? And there's nothing but my word to say it wasn't. But my word seems to count for shit, cos even Grace, my best friend in the whole goddamn world, even she doesn't seem to hear me.

From: Grace Ashdown   **Today 00:43**
To: Izzy Chambers
Re: us

even if ud pick up i don't even want 2 try 2 call u right now izzy just the sound of ur voice and i swear id proper flip

seriously wtf is going on?

we agreed

you promised

i don't ask much. i just wanted some time with Nell and u said ud say i was with u

is that what this is about? cos i have Nell? cos i cant see what else would make you act like this?!?!?! its proper mean izzy

ur supposed to be my best friend

all u had 2 do was say i was with u and mum wd have come home no questions asked

u with jacob? is that it? what kind of idiot are u? i mean jacob mansfield? how long has that been going on? since the party? is that why uv gone quiet on me?

mums gone proper mental. grounded me

daniel says uv gone away 4 a few days well u might want 2
stay there cos every1 knows what uv been up 2 with jacob

u didn't even say sorry

leave me alone 4 a bit

i mean it

grace

Grace and I never email. We message or we real-life talk and
that's it. Until now.

And there was Mum, when we were talking about who'd
have which bed, telling me she'd take the bottom bunk cos
'I'm probably being silly, Izzy, but I just feel I can protect you
better from down here.'

I tried to snuff all that better-late-than-never derision from
my nose. Anyway, fat lot of good she's done. She couldn't stop
the email, could she? No protection from that; no chance of
reconciliation either cos Mum and I are on verbal lockdown.
Anyway, Grace doesn't want an explanation even if I were
allowed to give it. *Leave me alone*, she said. *I mean it.* And
those words right there should probably be the most hurtful,
but the word I keep going back to is *Nell*.

Grace upper-cased it. The only time her fury could be
paused long enough to press the shift key on her MacBook was
when she thought of Nell. And I know, I know, I'm not
supposed to be the angry one here, but if it weren't for

Elizabeth's welcome speech and her multiple pleas to think of the other women and children, I mean it, I'd scream. That kind of wide-mouth-horror-movie scream that shatters windows.

Like it'd do any good. Cos even when I do make noise, like say sorry literally five times over, no one hears it. Not even Grace. So, honestly, there's no point in my words and no point in my screaming at all.

The house is as quiet as me. Not like Whitstable, gulls blasting from dawn and next door's cat on our decking, its meow like a baby given its first taste of ice cream, practically squealing this constant beg for more. Daniel goes out to it sometimes, whispers 'shoo' just loud enough so we can hear how gentle he's being. And he might think he's fooled me, but I know he hates cats, though maybe he just hated Sinitta because she belonged to me.

She didn't always. Belong to me, I mean. Before Sinitta was mine she was my dad's. He showed me a picture of her when he came to see me, said maybe I'd like to meet her one day.

The first time I saw her was the day of his funeral, when we went back to his parents' house and the sitting room was filled with grown-ups dressed in black. I only came up to their hips. Sinitta was under a table in the corner of the room, the exact same spot I'd have liked to have been in, so I crawled around ankles to get to her, leant against the wall with my hand stretched out until she came over and sat on my lap. The vibrations of her purr were just how my heart was feeling. We didn't move until everyone else had left and my dad's mum came over and told me there'd been some things in the boot of the car when Dad —

115

She couldn't say it. Not yet. But she gave me the necklaces, the record and the photo album, told me Dad had been so happy to know me. 'If only he'd found out sooner,' she said, and I didn't understand the look she gave my mum. Not then. I get it now. 'Sinitta obviously likes you.'

I was too busy getting the kitten to chase the necklaces to hear the conversation in which they decided the cat would be added to the box of all this new stuff I had to take home. I swear I thought it was the best party bag ever.

Sinitta never liked Daniel. Not that she'd hiss or anything – she'd simply pretend he wasn't there. He tried so hard at the beginning too, but for all his George Clooney charm, he couldn't persuade her to go anywhere near him. 'Stupid cat,' he'd say. I saw him kick her once, though obviously he wasn't really kicking her cos 'That would be cruel, Isabel, and I'm not cruel, am I? I tripped over her. The dumb animal was in my way.'

And he'd say she was ruining his garden and stinking his house out, but Sinitta wasn't like all our other things Daniel persuaded us to get rid of when we moved. No matter what he said, she was for keeps.

But then came the vom. And not just a bit of it. Like, a few times a day every day for a week, sending Daniel kind of batshit.

Then, just like that, she was gone.

It wasn't Daniel who arranged it either. I heard Mum on the phone, giving her name and our address and explaining we really couldn't keep Sinitta, and yes, she was a great cat and superb with children, so if they could find a new home that would be lovely.

'Lovely,' she said. And yeah, her voice was a violin, but she said it anyway. Lovely.

I tried to run away. Just me and Sinitta, who didn't much like being in my rucksack, her head poking through the open zip, but I carried on down the street in spite of the meows and the smell of that sick and I snapped. 'Please, Sinitta, that's what's got us into this trouble in the first place.'

'It's not your mum's fault, not really, but she can't cope with that cat.' It had taken Daniel hardly any time to catch up with me. 'She's finding everything very stressful at the moment, Isabel. You've got to be a good girl. Don't make things worse for her, please. Now give me the bag.'

And as her purr got louder and the vibrations got stronger, it felt like I was handing him my heart.

TWENTY-FIVE

It's 6:30a.m. and I've already left the refuge, no clue how I get back in but, whatever, cos it's not like I'm returning any time soon. Not that I'm running away or anything – history's proven I'm pretty crap at that! – but I've no desire to spend the day in there while Mum makes friendship bracelets and pinkie promises with her new BF Kate.

And seems I'm not the only one up with the crack of dawn. I'm barely even away from the house when there's a ping that I'm sure is gonna be Grace, cos the most we've ever gone without speaking is twelve hours and that was only because she had bird flu and her dad had run out of antibac wipes with which to sanitise her phone.

Please, Izzy. Can we talk?

Right message. Wrong sender. Max.

I delete it, cos what's the point? Focus instead on remembering which turns I've taken, until I come to this bridge that's like spending time with Daniel when you first cross it, how it looks like this safe passage over the water but actually it wobbles with every step. It feels steadier now I'm standing still in the middle, looking upriver where, from around the bend, comes this moving shape, a rower, their back to me, pulling themselves closer and closer with no clue even that I'm there. How can they do that? Trust their path without seeing it? Have that faith in themselves that, despite the blindness of the future, they'll be OK?

From the bulk of the body, it's a man: broad shoulders, pale arms, muscles bulging with the back and forth of the oars. His movement is so seamless, so clean, it makes it clear what kind of guy he is: fearless, determined, strong.

So maybe Grace was on to something then when, in the wake of all that fingers crap, she told me to stand tall. 'You know, Izzy, your body says *so* much about you.'

'I think we both know what *my* body says about *me*.'

'Nah-ah-ah.' She raised a waggy finger. 'That's what *Jacob* has *told* people about your body. *You* need to take matters into your *own* hands. I mean, *seriously*, Iz, it's not just the party – it's like in these last few months you've *literally* shrunk or something. Come *on*, head up.' That waggy finger lifted my chin. 'Shoulders back.' Grace's palms pulled me straighter from behind. 'Eighty percent of language is *physical*, babe. You don't even have to *say* anything – just let your goddamn *body* do the talking. Let your *don't give a shit, stand up, strut it out, walk on by, whole body acting like a middle finger* show them you couldn't care less about the crap Jacob Mansfield and his cronies are spreading. It's *gestures* that count. Not words.'

The words Daniel speaks are mostly kind, or would seem that way if I repeated them, like I did to Mum's friend Becky that time in town, or when I mentioned to Grace once that Daniel told Mum over and over how he'd never let her go.

'Sweet,' Grace had said, because the words alone were a lover's cliché.

Daniel's face though. Daniel's hands. They were a different story.

Grace was right then: the physical *is* greater than the spoken, our bodies have a tale of their own. Only, Mum's – after Daniel has said all that he's said and done all that he's done – well, Mum's body has become a closed book. Her cover's made of long sleeves and half-smiles and her title's something like *I'm Fine* or *He's Promised He'll Change* or *He's Just Passionate* even. But inside, her story is something else. Something like a glass slipper shattered into a hundred pieces on the floor.

The rower, he's the opposite of that. He's so together, so sure of himself. Where does that even come from? That confidence. That knowledge that your body will see you through. I *did* have it, I reckon, in those days on the grass outside the flat when I'd turn cartwheel after cartwheel, arms and legs mightier than the dizziness determined to topple me. Forward rolls too. Headstands and handstands, dress falling down over my face but no blush-cheeked rush to turn upright, to cover myself, to hide my belly or my thighs or any of those other parts of me which, only a few years later, were so readily blotted with shame. Mum on the bench with a mug of tea she'd brought down from the flat, calling scores out of ten, then lifting me on to the podium wall, where she'd offer up a Garibaldi biscuit to my chest like it was pure Olympic gold.

Those were the days, right? When I didn't care if my body was beautiful enough but if it was fierce enough, when the only wobble that worried me was the one before a fall.

The rower is closer now, and maybe not so much of a man as an almost grown-up like me. But so unlike me it almost hurts to look.

He *owns* that boat. It's under his will. Like I am with Jacob, I think, and I choke at the thought of the photos, of me beneath that body he owned as he took that body I hated. For what? For a chance of not being exposed as what everyone already knows I am. Something dirty and ruined and too buried beneath the shame of things to get even a slither of the sunshine or moon.

Another boat comes along, with four rowers and someone shouting at them when to pull, where to turn, but they still go wrong, their oars out of sync and their end in the bank. The lone rower seems so much calmer. More powerful. More in control.

And there's my answer, I reckon, and it's stupid that I've only just realised, because isn't the thing that most appeals about *Desert Island Discs* its isolation? I don't need to be cast away to an island. I need to *be* one. A rock. A lone rower making my own way through the water. No one else to bring me down.

Screw you, I send to Daniel.

Screw you, I send to Jacob.

Screw you, I send to Grace.

And I don't send it to Mum. But she'll know exactly how I feel.

The rower looks up just as he dips under the bridge and, like I'm playing Poohsticks, I run to the other side, where he reappears, face tilted towards me, and I lift my head up, pull my shoulders back and shout, 'Thank you', because in his solitude he's taught me how I might just stand a chance of owning my piece of the sky.

TWENTY-SIX

It smells. Not like gross or anything, but if you bottled it, put it in a line-up with bottles of other places, I could pick out the refuge for sure. It smells of bleach and tinned soup and conditioner on damp towels. Dove Intensive Repair. I swear from the shelf in the bathroom, all the women here must use it, like they think everything about them needs fixing, including their hair.

Mum's been at it too, towel like a bandage around her skull and her face like a wound when I walk in to find her sitting on the edge of the bed, bare legs poking out of her towel like she's chilling at some kind of spa.

'Why didn't you answer my calls, Izzy?' And I can't tell if the red of her cheeks is from the fix-up job in the shower or that noiseless anger she has, how it works its way out through her skin.

'I just wanted some space, all right.' I've only been back a few minutes and could already do with some more. The room is tiny; even though Mum brought me barely anything from Daniel's, we still fill it, with our bags and our bodies and all those unspoken words, those unfulfilled promises. And our shame.

It's like being back at home in that sense. At Daniel's, I mean. That place where shame settled like dust despite his ability back in the beginning to make us shine.

'Come on, Stephanie.' The air above the seat of our second-hand green chair became a galaxy of tiny stars as Daniel gave the cushion a theatrical smack. 'Do you really want this fusty old thing when we agreed we'd buy everything new?'

We were sorting the flat, packing up our first real home before moving in with Daniel. All but the living room done and he'd written *TO TAKE* on just three boxes. I knew Mum could feel my plea, I could see it in her fingers, how both thumbs were picking at the nails of both pinkies. After wiping the fusty old dirt from his palms, Daniel slipped his hands into hers and held them steady.

'Fresh start,' he said.

Mum looked at me, like, *he's right, Isabel*, and it was the first time I wished things had been different. Just a little bit. Just enough for us to take the green chair, which had held us steady on those *Desert Island* Sunday mornings before Daniel's hands turned up promising to do a better job.

'I can't afford new things,' Mum said, and Daniel had laughed because hadn't he told us already, this would be his treat, whatever we wanted, whatever we needed to make it feel like home.

'You think your mum deserves better than this grubby lump, don't you, Isabel?' And when he put it like that…'You do too,' he said, ruffling my hair like I'd seen dads do to their kids in the movies. 'You can pick out some things for your new bedroom if you like.'

So, the green chair went back to the charity shop from which we'd bought it those eight years before and we went with our three boxes into Daniel's house, where *happiness* was framed and hung on the wall as confirmation of how he made us feel.

Two days later, Grace and I hung out for, like, an hour in B&Q, where some guy on the paint counter rolled his eyes comically as we squealed over Citrus Tickle, Fiddlehead Fern and Lime Candy. 'Anyone would think those paint charts were photos of Justin Bieber the way you two are carrying on,' he said, winking the kind of wink I imagined my grandad would have given me if he hadn't wanted to give me away.

'I don't care about *Justin Bieber*.' I knew by the volume of Grace's voice what was coming. 'I'm a *lesbian*, you see.' Grace liked to drag the word out like it was an elastic band, stretching it wide and then flicking it in the face of whoever she was trying to shock.

But the sales guy just nodded, like, *whatever floats your boat, love*, and Grace huffed and puffed cos she got off on the drama of it back then when she didn't have a Nell to get off on it with for real.

We were hooked on the greens, totally convinced Ivy Pasture was the sophisticated look my bedroom needed to give me that *je ne sais quoi*. Grace, who was in the top set in French, reassured me that was a good thing.

A week or so later, Daniel, who'd asked me to make a note of the paint name, was waiting for me when I arrived home from school, this Tigger bounce in his step when he opened the front door with his George Clooney uniform tie hung over his shoulder. 'Come, come, come,' he said, everything turning to black as he wrapped the tie around my eyes and took my hand to guide me up the stairs. 'I was going to wait for your mum, but it's just too good.'

I'd never smelt fresh paint, never had that rush of fumes, that annihilation of everything that was there before. I must have held my nose or coughed or something because Daniel was telling me not to be such a baby, it wouldn't last long, and to think of him all those hours up the ladder, but wasn't it worth his effort because: 'ta-da!' And he tugged at the blindfold to reveal my new room painted an orangey red.

'But the green,' I said.

Daniel looked at me, like, *what?*

'Ivy Pasture!' I tried to use the 'indoor voice' he'd suggested when Grace had come over for the first time after we'd moved in the weekend just gone, but maybe I was still too loud, cos Daniel flinched as if my words had been hurled like stones.

'There's no need to shout at me, Isabel.'

'Sorry,' I said, 'but this isn't the colour I wanted.' I pulled the colour chart from my drawer. 'Ivy Pasture, see.'

'Oh.' His voice was like flat lemonade, still sweet but it had lost its fizz. 'My bad. This is *Autumn* Ivy. So close. I've spent all day on it too. Turned down an advert so I could get it done for you. I even ruined one of my favourite T-shirts.' The lines didn't disappear from his forehead when he rubbed it. 'Never mind. I can probably cancel that Clooney gig I've got next week – I could repaint it then. Your mum will be OK going without that sofa she had her heart set on.' He picked at the flecks of paint on his hands. 'I was going to use the cash from that job to get it for her, you see.'

'It's fine,' I said, even though the new colour was like brick, heavy and porous, soaking up all the good vibes – I mean, that was why Daniel was acting so weird, right?

'No, no.' He took the colour chart from me, fingered the Ivy Pasture. 'It's not at all fine, Isabel. I wanted everything to be perfect – that's why I spent so long on it. Why I got the best primer and was so careful with the edges. But if you don't like the colour —' It was left hanging, that 'if', like the *happiness* in the frame in the hallway depended on it.

'No, really.' The colour chart tore easily when I pulled it from him, crumpling the pieces into a tight ball. 'This is much nicer.'

'Attagirl,' Daniel told me.

When Mum asked me that evening why the change of heart, he gave me a conspiratorial nudge with his elbow, said we'd both realised, hadn't we, Isabel, that green wasn't the colour for me.

Maybe it was the paint, maybe it was Daniel's insistence that everything be put away each evening; that if it wasn't, he reserved the right to go into my room and tidy it himself. He did too.

'You should see it as a lesson, Isabel,' he said, chirpy as a CBeebies presenter. 'If you'd just kept it shipshape like I'd asked, I'd never have touched your record player.'

That didn't explain why he'd dropped it, why it had broken into too many pieces to play Dad's 'You Are My Sunshine', why Mum turned quiet and pink and said, 'It's fine, Isabel.'

The more I looked at her, the more I thought of how in our old flat the shapes of our bodies would stay bent into the cushions on the sofa; how she would find me sometimes by the trail of biscuit crumbs I'd left from the kitchen to my bed; how when it was just the two of us, things may have been messier, but they'd been so much warmer too.

So maybe it was the paint, or maybe it was those other things, those things which felt like nothing at the time, but whatever it was, that bedroom in Daniel's house was never really mine, like this one in the refuge isn't mine – ours – either.

'*It's fine, Izzy,*' as Mum would say, but even as the room feels full, there's so much missing. And I don't even mean my Jar of Sunshine, though that'd help. But walking in, finding Mum looking half relieved, half scared to shit, what hits me is that what we had in the flat, what we hadn't squeezed into those three boxes, was that quiet calm that comes with honest, uncomplicated love.

Our love, the honest and uncomplicated love I shared with Mum, was left behind when she was taken in by Daniel's. Mum let that love go. Mum *let* love – her love for Daniel – do this to her. She *let* Daniel's love take her into darkness while all the time she let her love for me do shit.

It's hot, this realisation. Like scorching embers in my belly threatening to erupt into fire, and I must jolt with the blaze of it or something, cos Mum looks up at me, pupils dilating into those familiar pools of fear, but even the whisper that if I screw her fear and blow like I'm sure I'm about to then I'm not so different from Daniel – even that doesn't stop me. And I can practically feel it then, that power I see in Daniel's eyes whenever I see that fear in Mum's.

'Why the fuck did you stay with him?'

It feels so good to finally scream it. To burn. And though

my cheeks are already wet from the shame of scaring her, I stand my ground, towering over my mother, ignoring the fact that she's weeping because I am an island and her tears will just wash away.

TWENTY-SEVEN

'I'm sorry' are the only words I can understand. The rest are choked in sobs and smothered by her hands on her face, which she can't bring herself to lift to me since I asked her the question surely anyone would ask if they knew.

'Why don't you come with me, Izzy?'

I buck the hand from my shoulder, turn to see Kate, whose concern is as clear as her bruises.

'We can make your mum a cuppa. One sugar, Steph?'

And they sound like proper friends already. *Bully for you*, I think, cos *they're* all right, aren't they, with their new mate bunking up in a room down the corridor while mine's over two hundred miles away and hates me to hell.

'This isn't the end of it, Mum.' If anything, my venom's more audible now I've quit shouting.

'It's the end of it for now,' Kate says as she steers me towards the kitchen, and her tone's like Ms Robinson's in school, the only female teacher even the boys didn't dare give shit to. 'Tea? Coffee?' She's suddenly softer, giving a smile when she pulls Elizabeth's biscuits from the very back of the cupboard. 'Secret stash,' she says, putting two on a small plate, sliding it towards me across the table.

It's funny, isn't it, the things that make you cry. How I barely even flinched when Daniel threw the still-burning

Yorkshire pudding tray at the back of Mum's head as she bent down to get the potatoes from the oven. How I stayed dead still and dead silent the time he took a fork and scraped it from her chest to her hips after he discovered she'd lied about what she'd eaten for lunch. 'This little piggy went to McDonald's,' he said. 'Did you really think I wouldn't find out?' She'd given up trying to pull her top down, hadn't even attempted to fend him off.

'Isabel should stay, Stephanie,' he said when she told me to go to my room. 'She needs to see how deceitful her mother is. Why it's so difficult for me to trust you, my wife, when you lie about such silly things as McNuggets.' He laughed then, not a big laugh, but caught my eye, shook his head and expelled a small puff of can-you-believe-this-woman laughter from his nose. I could believe it though because by then life seemed to have lost its element of surprise.

But my tears are a surprise now. The tears and the intake of breath at the tinny clatter of the plate's slight wobble as it slides across the table. The way the refuge kitchen becomes Daniel's kitchen and Kate becomes Daniel and the biscuits become the start of the trail of the last few days that led us here. It's a flash of a thing and it all disappears, of course, to the secret stash at the very back of my mind, the bit not even Grace has a key to, so Kate can think again if she reckons a Rich Tea and that smile she's smiling, that I-know-what-you've-been-through-cos-I've-been-there-got-the-T-shirt look she's wearing, has any hope of making me confess my darkest.

But surprise number two: she doesn't even try, just sits there as I work on being a rock, dry and deserted, pulling back the tears and filling my mouth with biscuits so it doesn't accidentally fill with words.

My phone vibrates in my pocket. And if I weren't an island, I'd scrabble for it, right? My heart would pump with the hope of Grace Grace Grace. And it might panic too, that if my *screw you* was a volcanic eruption then this reply is a tsunami wave. But I sit. I eat my second biscuit. I thank Kate for my tea and I leave. As quiet and calm as the lone rower. In complete control.

It's only when I'm outside that I let myself look at the message, and I can't help it, how my heart crashes when it's not Grace but Daniel. How I can't not feel scared of him despite my island guard.

Screw you? That's a little unkind, Isabel. I realise I'm not your real dad, but I want your life to be filled with sunshine just as much as he did. Your mother's too. Let me know where you are and I can drop this over to you x

Attached is a photo of my Jar of Sunshine. If the picture were of a human, I'd half expect the person to be bound and gagged or clutching a sign with details of the ransom: *Tell Daniel everything or the jar gets it.*

'Bad news?' I hadn't expected Kate to follow me out into the garden.

I tilt the screen away, stand tall.

'You know Elizabeth can arrange for you to speak with a counsellor.'

Here she goes – I knew the quiet wouldn't last long.

'Or maybe chatting with some of the other girls who've stayed here with their mums might help.'

But I don't want a counsellor or other girls. If I did want to speak with anyone, which obviously I don't, then there's only one girl I'd want it to be.

'Izzy, love.'

Anyone who didn't know Mum would think she sounded normal, but her voice is a tiptoe. She stands before me on the patio, next to Kate, who puts a hand on the small of her back, becomes her stabiliser, just like that. Nothing to it but a small gesture to show that she's there.

I'd like to do the same, honestly I would. I'd like to go to my mum and hold her, tell her I'm OK, she's OK, being here's OK and we'll move on. But sometimes embers don't grow into fire and beyond the silence and biscuits, we can't do anything at all.

TWENTY-EIGHT

You'd think a refuge might be brimming with sadness but, turns out, laughter's kind of normal in a place like this, especially among the kids, whose stomps on the stairs give away heavy-footed clues in their games of hide-and-seek. The irony of the hunt's not lost on me, but the children squish themselves into wardrobes and under beds, totally into the idea of somebody chasing them down.

It's safe when it's a game. When it's here in this house that's not theirs, not ours. No one can touch us.

But Jacob's tried. In the message he sent on Sunday night, he said he's waiting. Said I have a fortnight's grace because when he went round to check on me, Daniel told him I'm away with my gran.

What do you think your gran would say, Fingers, if she saw her precious little Izzy like this? Two weeks, remember. Tick tock.

But time is safe here too. There is no college. There is no timetable. There is no Daniel tapping his watch, reminding Mum she needs to be in bed before ten. There is space between the minutes to breathe. And when they're not working or figuring out the rest of their lives, Mum and the other women here drink tea and read the papers in the sitting room, where they chat about last night's telly, the Brexit cock-up and

Trump's most recent crass comment. They make lunch, snacks and dinner and call out to the children that if they hurry, they might just squeeze in a quick trip to the park before bath and bed. Kate is the only one with a bruised face; none of the others – there are three of them – look like they belong here. I wonder if we do.

We're not exactly getting on – we're getting by. There are forms to fill. Decisions to make. Money to find. We get further with some things than others. Some, like the baby, aren't mentioned at all. If it was the death of Daniel's mother that sent us back to him the last time, maybe its opposite, the birth of his child, might do the same now. So we keep quiet. But Mum suggests we 'talk to someone together'. She doesn't specify about who or what, though I'm guessing it's all the stuff we don't manage to talk about when it's just the two of us. My refusal sits in my belly like too much mashed potato. A heavy lump of stodge that gets worked off on my walks to the river so I swear I feel lighter and more willing when I'm there, more like I'm gonna go back to the refuge and be kind to my mum, who's trying so hard to make things better. And I'll give her a chance, I think, when my toes are dipped in the water, but then I get near her, and the sunshine slips away.

'I've got this appointment.' Her voice is a child balancing on a log with a nervously held out hand.

And I'd take it, but I think about all those times when *I* could have done with some propping.

She pulls at the ends of her hair, which is loose around her shoulders, the only way Daniel likes it.

'Honestly, Stephanie,' he'd said, 'it's as if you think you're seventeen with all these ponytails and plaits. I hate to break it to you –' he kissed the nape of her neck – 'but the time for those styles was your knocked-up teenager years.' He was laughing, not scornful but friendly, the soft teasing kind, when he twisted her round so they were head to head. 'You're so beautiful though, especially with your hair long. And down,' he added, before sliding the hairband from her pony-tail and tossing it into the bin.

'So this appointment,' she says. 'It's —'

'I'm going to the river,' I tell her.

Even though I'm this rock, it hurts to push her away.

'Sure,' she says, already giving up, which further rallies the storm in me, cos if she only persevered a little longer…'Keep your phone with you.'

'I love you so much, Izzy,' she says when I get to the door from our bedroom to the hallway. The crack in her voice trying so hard to be like the split in the meringues we used to bake in the flat. All gooey in the middle, but at the bottom reliably firm.

She bends when she holds me, her back rounding as her arms stretch wide around my middle, hands like she's gather-ing in the loose parts of me, my nose caught in her under-repair hair as she says it again and again. 'I love you, Izzy. I love you, Izzy. I love you.'

I hate it, how my bones soften and begin to yield to the warmth of her, how the anger that runs through my spine starts to topple like those skinny Lego-brick towers I'd build as a kid, big chunks of it crashing down to the floor. But I catch them before it's too late, stack them back up again, these rigid spites of mine, make them into a shape that can stand on its own two feet. And I go.

Leaving gives me a chance to look at the messages I've kept hidden from Mum. None from Grace. Only that one from Jacob. It's Daniel who's been busiest. More pictures of my Jar of Sunshine, which he's positioned round the house like that stupid Elf on the Shelf Grace was so into at Christmas a few years back.

In one, Daniel has my Jar of Sunshine in the biscuit tin, which he's filled with my favourites. No expense spared – they're those super-thick milk chocolate rings, those ones in the Tesco Chocolate Biscuit Assortment, four quid a box and there are only two of each type in every pack. There's got to be, like, thirty of the buggers in the picture, arranged in a perfect circle around the jar, with a yellow Post-it to match the yellow beads: *A sweet treat for my sweet girls' homecoming…*

Then there's the jar held up in front of a screen filled with the Netflix logo, another Post-it stuck to the edge of the TV: *All ready for the perfect night in. The only thing missing is…you.*

I'd begged Mum for Netflix – everyone at college was talking about *Pretty Little Liars* and *13 Reasons Why* and it hadn't been so bad before Nell, when I could live, like, seventy percent of my life at Grace's, where we'd sprawl on her bed, our attempts at nail art inevitably screwed by our heads cricked up to the TV drama and crumbs from our snacks slipping into the wet varnish. Then along came Nell. And my time with Grace was, like, halved and I didn't want to spend it not talking, even if Grace did talk mostly about Nell's impression of Ariana Grande – side-splitting, apparently

– Nell's smile – mesmerising – and Nell's kisses – heaven. Maybe I should have stuck with the TV.

Anyway, I asked Mum for Netflix, but she stopped work three years ago when Daniel said it was taking too much of her time away from me: 'Don't you need her now more than ever, Isabel, what with your GCSEs on the horizon? And it's such an important age, as you well know, Stephanie.' He'd paused then, this long look from Mum to me. 'It's so easy for things to go wrong.' And she wasn't to worry financially because Daniel had that inheritance money, and they could sell Mum's car if she wasn't working. It would only be for a few years. 'It's nothing in the grand scheme of things,' he'd said. 'You want to put Isabel's needs before your own, don't you?' Mum nodded, like, *sure*, even though she loved her new position at the bank and even though without her income, it was no longer up to her if we had Netflix or went to the cinema or bought new clothes, because everything had to be run by Daniel, who rolled his eyes and said hadn't she thought of all this when she decided to quit her job, hadn't she realised the burden she'd be placing on him, and wasn't he doing his best, and sorry, but, no, Netflix wasn't a priority right now, when times were tough, what with the acting work not going so well and the Clooney bookings being down since the arrival of 'that bitch Amal'. Of course he'd laughed then, because he'd never really talk that way about a woman – 'I'm just not that kind of guy.'

Memories, eh.

And Daniel's full of them. Because along with the daily Jar of Sunshine pictures are the daily ones of the three of us, in Paris or London, or today his house, the time he decorated it with fairy lights and a tepee after he ripped up Mum's ticket to Glastonbury a couple of years back. I wasn't sure what to do when he'd asked me to help him; it was as if heaving those monolith rocks he'd had delivered so he could make our very own stone circle would make me complicit in the scenes that had come before. 'Please, Isabel.' His head was cocked to one side, that George Clooney grin broad and so damn sure I'd cave in. 'Your mum will be a nightmare if you don't. You know how she gets when she thinks she's missing out. That temper! I can't do it on my own.' And his George Clooney eyes took over from his George Clooney mouth. 'Please.'

It was actually pretty fun while it lasted. We wore fairy wings and wellies, and Daniel painted butterflies on our faces. 'You're both so beautiful,' he said. 'My princesses.' And I wondered if this *was* better than Glastonbury because, like Daniel kept pointing out, we had all of the music and none of the mud. 'And you didn't have to leave me behind,' he said to Mum as she sipped on her water because Daniel thought she'd probably had enough beer for one day. 'Who needs a soggy field and their friends,' he said, 'when you have your husband and your daughter and this?' He spread his arms, turning in circles around the garden, where we'd hung lanterns and pitched a tent. 'Sometimes, Stephanie, you need to be more grateful for what you have in your home with the people who love you most. And, my god, do we love you!' His voice was like the candyfloss we'd made for the food stall in the kitchen.

We're wearing headdresses in the photo he sent this morn- ing. And smiles. We look happy. Really happy. I remember showing it to Grace, who was totally in awe of the efforts Daniel had gone to. 'God, Iz, my dad is *so lame* by comparison. So *suburban*. I swear the best thing he's done for my mum is, like, *mow the lawn* into those stripes she likes so much. Daniel's just *so* much more thoughtful. Your mum is *so* lucky.'

'*Why the fuck did you stay with him?*' I'd screamed.

Well, I guess Mum thought the same as Grace sometimes. We both did.

TWENTY-NINE

Like most days since I've been here, I head for the river, which is weird, right, cos the sea's always been my thing – Grace and I would stand on the groynes with one hand to our forehead like we were some kind of sea captain, in awe at the giant mass of it. A river, pah! A river was merely a thing that might lead you to the ocean. It was never the main event. It was a warm-up.

And lie-ins were my thing too. But mornings, like everything else, are different here. There's this baby who wakes at, like, 6:17 on the dot, screaming out for her mother like they're shacked up in different wings of a mansion, not sleeping, like the rest of us, in the 'family rooms', a maximum of three foot apart.

So every day I'm up, no point competing for the bathroom cos the kids are all desperate for a wee and the mums are all desperate for a dollop of Intensive Repair so I leave them to it. Meanwhile, *my* mum, who's always been up and at 'em early, only quietly obviously so as not to wake Daniel, who needs his beauty sleep, you know, what with being a Clooney lookalike and all – well, here *my* mum manages to sleep through whatever kind of hell is breaking loose, which seems to happen most mornings when some kid's Weetabix is too soggy, or one of the mums can't find her phone. Usually turns out a kid who may or may not be her own is using it to hard-line episodes of *Peppa Pig*. I don't stick around for the come-down, walking instead to the river, where I stand on the bridge, all casual, like, not waiting for anyone, definitely not looking for oar-shaped ripples in the water cos that'd be, like, totally lame, and I'm totally not lame any more. I'm a rock, remember.

And even though I'm definitely not waiting, definitely not looking, every morning I see him, that lone rower. And I swear the only reason I get this tingle is absolutely nothing to do with how cute he is and everything to do with him being a reminder of why it's better to be alone.

But despite my best efforts at being a bit more hermit, in my head there's all this music careening between Katy Perry's 'Teenage Dream', Wrathschild's 'Fall into Love' and Ray LaMontagne's 'You Are the Best Thing'. And even though I'm one hundred percent rock, I might sometimes listen to these tracks on my way to the bridge *and* when I'm on the bridge, so pretty much all that time in the morning when I'm definitely not waiting and definitely not looking, I listen and, goddamn that lone rower because, yeah, yeah, I'll admit it, I'm close to a literal swoon.

But anyway, it's lunchtime, so no chance of swooning, and in any case, turns out, as I absolutely already knew, Rower Boy's not the only thing I like about the river. Maybe it's the way it cuts up and connects things, or how the ducks are so easily carried along in its flow, or that the kids of the town seem equally drawn to it. There are eight of them, five boys, three girls, sitting on the bank in front of the boathouse, the bare-chested guys flinging themselves and each other into the water while the girls remain dry, watching on.

I sit on the opposite bank with a Starbucks grande hot chocolate even though it's, like, twenty-seven degrees. Two of the group don't even bother to sidle off before kissing, totally at ease with each other's bodies, his hand holding her cheek, her leg crossed over his thigh. Despite the others milling about, the moment seems so gentle, so in tune with the lazy summer and the quiet run of the river. The opposite of everything I've known. Everything I've felt. I can't take my eyes off them, my curiosity matched by my envy of how unlike me they are, the effortlessness with which they sink into each other, how she doesn't suck herself in, shrink herself back, and how their kiss seems as endless as the water, until the rest of the lads start rapping, bringing the kissing boy out of his moment and into this pack of modern-day poets wooing their girls with their words.

Only, the harder I listen, the clearer it is that they're not. Wooing, I mean. What they *are* doing is chanting, egging each other on with this song that honestly can't be but literally *is* about rape. Five boys stand on a riverbank in broad sunlight singing about kicking, licking and raping someone's little sister. The girls sit back – maybe they've heard it before, cos they're as un-enraged as the dog walker who stops, and I think he's gonna say something, but he's only tying his laces before moving on, his expression unchanged by the line about whorish mothers touting for willy in London.

When one of them messes up, they start over, gathering closer like sportsmen hunkering shoulder to shoulder for a pep talk on taking the other team down. The girls chat among themselves, like this is normal, like it's OK for their mates, their boyfriends even, to talk like this, cos maybe it's just bants, right? Maybe it doesn't do any harm to say these things. Maybe sticks and stones may break our bones, but words will never hurt us.

Thing is, I'm not so sure, because those embers, they're back and proper flaming, stoked by the words and searing the insides of me with their hate. It's a full-on human-combustion kind of anger, my blood too hot to quench it, pumping it instead around the whole of me, and I swear if I did like the boys and jumped in the river, that too would be on fire, carrying me and this violent inferno all its hundreds of miles to the sea.

I wonder if they'd even notice. If those boys or the dog walkers would sense the change in current and the rising heat, or whether my boiling rage would be doused as the likes of Jacob Mansfield and Daniel Chambers leered from their sail-boats. *'It's a laugh, innit. Natural, innit. Seriously, Isabel, you're just a prude.'*

I swear I'm gonna jump in, swim over and scream, but the river seems noisier, fiercer, and is holding so much more beneath its surface than I'd imagined from the bridge, from where it had looked like a harmless flow. It's not so different from the boys in that sense. It's too big a battle. Because the boys' rap is just part of it, right? Daniel and Jacob too. Whatever it is that makes rape a laughing matter, that makes their song palatable for the people passing by, that makes the girls not stand up and tell their mates to fuck off and never talk to or touch them again, it's just one part of something so much greater than five lads on a grassy bank singing about breaking a woman's spine. So maybe Grace was on to something when she bothered to go march against Trump. Maybe she was right to tell me I needed to speak up. Cos maybe it's all the same thing. Whatever it is that gave Jacob the right to do what he did. Whatever it is that gave Daniel the strength to do what he does with *his* words and *his* hands and *his* power that he wraps around Mum and me like a net in his water. Whatever it is, this greater thing they're part of, it's like the river, cutting up and connecting things, working its way through our cities and countryside until it reaches the Celtic Sea, the Atlantic Ocean, all the way to America, where a man who became president has made pussy-grabbing fair game.

Those embers? They're not just lit – they're wildfire. There's a fervour in them. In me.

I'd thought Grace was playing superhero to the world instead of being a friend to me. And I'd thought Mum was overreacting when she shed actual tears the morning we woke to news of a victorious Trump, when she made me toast and tea and whispered, 'Don't ever let any man, even the most powerful man in the world, make you believe you're anything less than brilliant.' I'd thought she was a hypocrite, because why slate the president when it's your husband that beats you? And I'd thought she was melodramatic because he's over there and we're over here. It seemed so distant. But I get it now, how it cuts up and connects things.

And yeah, I must look like the mad one here, with the heat risen to my face and to my palms even, which are up in the air waving at those kids across the river. '*How can you?*' This volume doesn't feel like it belongs to me. '*Stop!*' And they look at me, like, *what?*, chins bucked at the gall of it, of this crazy bitch on the other side of the river calling them out on their fun.

'We got a touchy one,' the kisser hollers. 'On the blob, are you?'

If I was, I swear I'd pull the tampon from my vagina and sling it in his smug little face.

And then: 'Hey.'

But it's a calm hey, a friendly hey, a hey that comes from over here instead of over there. I hear that, I sense the difference in tone, and when I turn around, hands still in the air like I just might really, really care, I see it too, I spot the difference in how he sees me.

Trouble is, Rower Boy might be good, but his timing's bad, and the 'hey' I bark back at him is licked with the flames of my rage.

THIRTY

'You all right?'

A week ago, an hour or so ago even, the kindness in Rower Boy's voice would have been enough to put a lid on the inferno in my belly. His smile would have cut off the oxygen at source, replacing it instead with weak knees and butterflies. That literal swoon. But right now, that rap, those boys, my stepdad, Jacob's photos, his 'deal', my entire bloody life, is all the heat, fuel and oxygen my anger needs to burn, burn, burn. And so despite Rower Boy's gentle hand on my shoulder, maybe even a little because of it, I shout *No*, my temper coming at him fast and furious, the sparks of my outrage searing his concern and turning him a flustered kind of red.

'Sorry,' he says, backing off a little. 'I was only trying to help.'

And I'm sure he is and I'm sure he was, but he's one of them, isn't he? One of the fifty percent. And a stranger. I couldn't even trust the man who married my mum. How could I trust this boy? His smile may be bright, and his words may be right, but Daniel was a true Prince Charming who scorched that fairy-tale rescue of his princesses to dust.

Across the river, the lads are still at it.

'I'd steer clear if I were you, mate,' one of them bawls.

But when I turn around to go at them again, the girls are thrusting the boys' T-shirts at their bared pecs, pulling at their arms, like they've finally had enough. It's the girls' heads that are hanging though, as if they're the ones who should feel ashamed. '*Good riddance*,' I want to shout at all of them as they climb the hill and merge into the trees, but it seems old Izzy, quiet Izzy, wouldn't-say-boo-to-a-goose Izzy is back, so instead I just watch as the flames die down to a smoulder.

Because it turns out, the one thing sure to dampen the fire is my own tears. I hadn't even realised they were falling, but by the time I've dropped to the ground, head in my hands, my top is already wet from the stream of them.

Rower Boy doesn't say anything, but I know he's still there. Years of not seeing Daniel, of purposefully looking the other way, have given me that heightened sense of someone's breathing, of someone's stare.

We stay like this for a while, until a woman's voice cuts into his silence and my heaving mess of a cry. 'Everything OK?' she asks. 'I can wait with you while this young man leaves if you want.'

And I see what this must look like, as if Rower Boy's the one who's done this to me, cos maybe the kind female stranger is aware of the cutting up and connecting things too. But I can't let Rower Boy take the blame for the Rapper Boys' assault, and so I lift my head and tell her, honestly, everything will be OK.

'If you're sure then,' she says, walking away but swinging her head round to check on me three times before she disappears from view.

'I'm sorry,' I say without really thinking about it, because apologies are what Mum and I do when the temperature's chilled and we're brushing the ashes beneath the carpet so we can move on.

But Rower Boy looks at me like, *cool*, like it's not unusual for a girl to scream then collapse into tears at his *hey*. Like it really doesn't matter that, after days of definitely not waiting and definitely not looking but definitely waving and definitely smiling, in our first up-close encounter, I burst into a great ball of flames.

'They're dicks,' he says.

And I nod, relieved not to be shouting but wondering what happens next, not with Rower Boy – though, yeah, if I'm honest, I guess there's a part of me thinking about that too – but, with that all-body anger fading, what happens next with my life?

I hadn't known she was in me, that girl who won't stand for it, that girl who won't sit quietly on the sidelines while those boys flaunt their god-given 'right' to say and do what they want with our bodies. Where's she been all these years? All those times Daniel trampled, emotionally and literally, on my mum – where was she then? Where was her not-afraid-to-use-it voice? That strength to say stop when something is wrong? Because those things weren't there when I really needed them, when it was personal, when Jacob Mansfield thrust me against a radiator, threatened me into lying down on his monument bed, playing that hardcore and assuming I was up for whatever those men did to those women because everyone knows you can do anything, 'grab 'em by the pussy' if you want, cos that's what we're here for, right? For them. Why has it taken this long for her to bust through my timid little shell?

But better late than never, I reckon, going easy on myself for the first time in, like, years, because maybe this isn't all on me, maybe I'm not the one who needs to say sorry. And though she's no longer raging, I can feel her, this galvanised Izzy, twisting and turning like a new kind of river is running through my blood.

'They are,' I say. 'Dicks, I mean. Mega dicks.'

And Rower Boy smiles that smile and I smile too, cos after weeks, months, years of keeping quiet, it's good to be saying things aloud.

'That song,' he says, 'is it for real?'

When I Google the lyrics on my phone, it literally is. 'Some twelve-year-old,' I tell him.

And we stand, breath-on-the-neck close, watching the YouTube video of this kid whose head is shaking as he stumbles through – and sometimes forgets – the words, like he totally gets the offence in them, but screw it, he'll rap and record them anyway, cos what harm can it do? It's just YouTube. It's just words. It's just rape. Sticks and stones, yeah?

'Like you said.' Rower Boy turns to face me when it's played. 'A mega dick.'

'I've discovered they're not so rare,' I say, and for once I know exactly what I'm doing, challenging Rower Boy to prove he's not one of their kind.

THIRTY-ONE

'So if you're tough enough to take on the mega dicks, I reckon you're tough enough to take on the water.' We're approaching the bridge, Rower Boy nods at the river below.

It feels kind of odd, to be standing with him on the exact same spot where I've been definitely not looking and definitely not waiting for him each morning.

'Tough? Me?'

'Mega tough!' he says, brows raised, like, *why would you even question it?* 'I went to school with a couple of those mega dicks and no one ever really stood up to them. We could do with a few more of your kind round here.'

'My *kind*?'

'Yeah,' he says, voice like a round of applause, 'you know, the kind that don't take any shit.'

'You mean, the kind that don't take any shit and then burst into tears!'

'True. They did issue a flood warning when you really got going!'

'Ha ha.' I try not to smile too much, cos I'm an island, remember, and anyway, Rower Boy's on trial.

We stand side by side, shoulders touching, and all the time I'm telling myself the only reason for feeling so wobbly is the other people walking across the bridge, nothing to do with

Rower Boy, who asks in a voice which is all soft and whirly and not totally unlike the Mr Whippy ice creams those kids are stuffing into their faces in the park, 'What's with your accent? You're not from round here then?…Where are you staying?…How long are you here for?…What are you up to tomorrow?'

That last one is the chocolate flake! I try not to bite too soon.

'A few things planned.' I'm as vague as I was with his other questions, figuring as I already bared so much when I screamed wildfire at the rappers on the riverbank, maybe I should hold back on the finest of my mixed-up family. But seriously, there must be a train chugging through my chest or something, cos, what with the thump and the rumble, I swear I can hardly breathe.

'How about it then?' Rower Boy says, and I must look at him, like, what?, cos he points at the river. 'You know, that thing you're obviously so obsessed with! I mean, that's why you've been here on the bridge every morning, isn't it? To watch me.' He smiles this wicked smile. 'I mean, to watch *people* row?!'

'Actually, it's the quiet I'm obsessed with. You rowers tend to ruin that.'

'I can only apologise,' he says. 'And the only way to make it up to you is to give you a lesson. Six A.M. tomorrow, yeah? It'll be nice and quiet then. Just how you like it.'

He's almost back on solid ground before I think to ask where we should meet.

'Right here.' He gestures with both hands first at the bridge and then at me. 'Actually, right there. That exact spot you're in now. Where it all began!'

And I can't help it, I smile so hard my head might literally explode into tiny pellets of sunshine.

'I don't even know your name,' I shout as he makes to run up the hill.

'Harry. Like Styles, but without the tats.' He raises his arms to declare his un-inked skin. 'Or the millions,' he says, pulling out his empty pockets. 'Or the looks.' And I've never seen anyone pull off such a good impression of a sad-face emoji.

'Story of my life,' I call out, imagining Grace's face if she ever gets to hear about the time I pulled out a One Direction pun in my feeble efforts at flirting.

THIRTY-TWO

I know, this rowing thing is, like, the worst idea ever. It's only going to end badly, right? For medicine, I listen to a sad songs playlist on Spotify, all this light-quenching Tom Odell, Damien Rice, Amy Winehouse and Joni Mitchell to suppress my ridiculous flutterings to the concept of love. Because if my heart, like the rest of me, is already broken, isn't it safer, less painful, to keep all my broken pieces in the dark?

So before I'm even back at the refuge, I'm totally cured of all those inappropriate feels. Love is totally, one hundred percent, absolutely not on my to-do list. And never, ever will be. Romantically anyway. What I *am* more open to, love wise, is Mum. I dunno, maybe it'll fade like it usually does when I see her, but I'm not so sure. Because that river rage, it let something out or switched something inside me, opened my eyes to this bigger picture. And it's not like I've suddenly got it all figured out, but maybe this rock thing's not so wise. Maybe we're better fighting together and against than fighting alone and between. And Mum *did* leave. She may have waited a while, but she *did* leave – despite everything he said and did, she left. She took me from that house and that man and led me towards the sky.

It's Kate I see first when I return. Kate and her bruises, which have turned from purple to green. I wonder if it hurts when the lines that form round her eyes as she gives me this big grin cut into the puffiness, but she's all 'Steph! Izzy's here'. No wincing, just this nervy excitement that makes me want to bolt back out the door and wait all night by the river for Harry.

'Baldy baldy bandicoot,' sings this little girl – Ava, I think her name is – running into the kitchen, holding up her hands for this clapping game she taught me at the crack of dawn this morning.

Mum comes in after, beaming, with her head held high, more oval than I've ever seen it.

'Izzy,' Ava says, 'pleaaaaaaaaase.' She pushes my arms up into the start position, but they stay there, in jazz hands, incapable of clapping, cos god forbid Mum mistakes the noise for a round of applause.

'What the —'

'Izzy, Ava's right here.' Kate shoots me a stop-right-there warning to censor whatever inappropriate words might spew from my dropped jaw.

'But seriously, what the actual …'

Mum runs her hand over the smooth skin of her head, no self-consciousness in it, just this, like, appreciation of its newness or something. 'You hate it,' she says, but in a voice that clearly doesn't give a shit if I do.

'You've shaved it!'

'Yep.' Her face is like Grace's whenever she bunks off college to spend an afternoon kissing Nell at the beach huts. Like, *what of it?*

I so want to be cool with this. It's only hair, right? It's still my mum, there's just a bit less of her; she's just a bit shinier around the edges is all. But it's so extreme. It's so bald.

'You want to feel?' She comes closer, reaching out for my hand, raising it gently to her crown. I wonder what the hell is going on beneath the skin.

'I can't go back,' she says, and I shrug my shoulders, shake my head, like, *what?* And she takes both my hands in hers then gives a quick glance at Ava, who Kate coaxes from the room with the promise of Connect Four. 'This means I can't go back.'

And maybe I'm stupid, but I still don't get it, so Mum sits me down at the table, face like when she told me about the birds and the bees.

'He'd kill me.' Her voice is a newsreader's, serious and matter of fact. 'You know what he's like.' And I nod because, well, Mum and me, we're the only ones who do. 'Before, when we left the last time, I made you promises, Izzy. This time, I'm determined to keep them. This,' she says, pointing at her naked skull, 'it's my promise. Can you imagine what he'd do if he saw me like this?' She can't stop touching it. 'He'd go crazy, Izzy.' And there's no hesitation in my name, which seems to come naturally now that her voice is more like her own, not her recent own, but her green-chair-days own, her run-the-world own. 'You know how he liked my hair a certain length, a certain colour. Anything else was – how did he put it? Unacceptable.'

'You could've got a perm.' And I'm trying to be funny, obviously, but neither of us laughs.

'I think this is more of a statement, don't you!' And she

gives me this smile I hadn't realised I'd missed. 'I actually quite like it. How it makes me look so different. Kind of strong.' She looks younger, and those windows to her soul, they're brighter and more fixed on me too. None of these head-down, not-now, shame-filled glances in another direction. Like me by the river, she's standing her ground. 'You know what he'd call it?'

'What?'

'Disobedient.'

She's right. He'd take one look and ask her why she felt the need to disobey him. God knows what he'd do then.

We sit like this, kind of basking in her rebellion, my hand holding hers, me looking at her head but not really seeing it, seeing instead the last six years that led us here: a margherita pizza, a table of cake, a card filled with promises, the Eiffel Tower, dancing at the harbour while bearing a ring, the torn arm of a wedding dress, the whispered apologies, the kisses and a necklace of sunshine scattered on the floor. The raised voices, the hushed voices, the I-love-you-more-than-anything voices. The tea in bed, the festival at home, the holding gently, the pulling roughly, the whispered apologies and the sobbing that was his and not hers. The gifts for no reason, the raised hands for no reason, the leaving, the returning, the whispered apologies, the shame and the hate. She's come through it all.

'It's actually pretty badass,' I say. 'And brave.'

Mum holds me tight.

In my head, there's Grace: '*You don't even have to* say *anything – just let your goddamn body do the talking.*' And so I hold Mum even tighter back, letting her know exactly what I think of her and that shiny head of hers. What's done is done and this is the new her. The new us. We might not know exactly where we're going, but it's not backwards. It's not to him. Wherever it is, I think, our love will take us there. The love that makes us strong.

THIRTY-THREE

'You grab that end.'

'But this is huge. It's gotta be for two people, right? Can't I go out on my own?'

'You're kidding? You know how much trouble I'd get into if I let a novice out on a single. Sorry, but this morning you're stuck in a double with me!' And he actually winks. Like, proper shuts his left eye, cocks his head and makes that weird clicking sound people who wink make when they're actually winking.

'Can you not?'

'Can I not what? Wink?' And he winks again. 'What?' Harry's voice is an oar in the water, stirring things up. 'You don't like that?' So he does it again, obviously. And again. And then all the way down to the jetty, which is good, really, cos maybe if he's got one eye closed most of the way he'll be less likely to notice how puffed I am just lugging the bloody thing, and I haven't even started rowing yet.

'It's sculling, actually,' Harry says when I ask when he first started rowing.

'Huh?'

'What we're doing – it's sculling.'

'Oh, that's what we're doing, is it? Sculling?'

'What else would we be doing, Izzy?' And he can't help it, can he? He winks again, silently this time, with this giant grin across his face which I know he'd say isn't as cute as Harry Styles's but...

'Nothing. Like you said, we're just sculling.' I'm glad for the fact that my back's to him as I climb into the boat – it makes me bolder, I guess. 'Definitely not flirting.'

'God, no,' Harry says, his voice like those lines people get round their eyes when they smile. 'Definitely not that. And definitely not wondering whether you're single.'

'No. That'd be awful, right? But I am, even though you're definitely not wondering. I am. Single, I mean.'

'Good to know. Had I been wondering, which I definitely wasn't. But if I was, that would definitely be good because I'm definitely single too.'

'I wasn't wondering.'

'Obviously.'

'But if I were.' And maybe this not facing someone is the answer. I swear this kind of talk's never come so easily. Or maybe it's the river – like yesterday, when it released that wild tongue in me.

Do not even think about wild tongue right now, Izzy.

'Woaaaahhhh!' And Harry's hands are in full body contact with my shoulders as he climbs in and the boat rocks and I'm one hundred percent sure we're going in. 'Sorry 'bout that,' he says, when the boat comes to a wobbly kind of peace on the water.

'Should I be worried, Harry? I mean, you're supposed to be the expert here, and yet I – the "novice", I think it was you called me – managed to get in the boat without nearly drowning us in the process.'

'It was all that definitely not flirting.'

My skin's kind of tingling from where his palms have been.

'You got me a bit Stevie Wonder there for a moment,' Harry says.

'Blind?!'

'No, "Knocks Me Off My Feet"!'

And my back or my still-tingling shoulders must be, like, *what?*

'The song?' Then he only goes and sings it. Terribly, but perfectly terribly if you know what I mean. 'Sorry,' he says. 'It's top of my rom list.'

'Your what?'

'My rom list.'

'As I said before, your what?'

'My rom list, Izzy. You know, romantic playlist?' And he sounds it out really slowly like I'm some kind of moron who obviously should have assumed a hot rower in Shropshire would have a romantic playlist topped by Stevie Wonder's 'Knocks Me Off My Feet'.

'You have a romantic playlist?'

'Yeah, what of it? I spend my life on the river – I'm bound to be soppy.'

I grin so hard I swear the glee in it will cause some kind of refraction in the sunlight on the water.

'Don't judge me, Izzy. I have playlists for every occasion. There's the rom list, the rage list, the Monday morning list, the I Can't Stand My Parents list and, of course, the XXX list.'

There's a kaleidoscopic flash of Jacob's laptop, the XXX list of videos he had on there.

'You all right, Izzy?'

'Huh? Yeah, I'm good,' I say, feeling a surge in the embers as I imagine chucking that MacBook in the Severn. 'Just thinking I might need an I Can't Stand Mega Dicks list.'

'Ha! Those mega dicks could rap their rap and we could play our list louder and prouder on the opposite bank.'

'*Our* list?'

'Well, I didn't mean to be presumptuous but —'

'Let's see how well this morning goes before we commit to a joint list, Harry. I mean, that's serious stuff! Come on, let's row.'

'Scull, Izzy! Let's scull!'

'Whatever,' I say, hoping it's not just the river because I want this feeling everywhere. 'Go on then.' I dare to turn around and smile. 'Tell me what I've got to do.'

So he does, and I try, and I'm not totally fall-in-the-water kind of rubbish, just oars-bashing-into-my-knees kind of clumsy.

'Blades!' Harry says. 'You keep calling them oars, but they're blades.'

'They're bloody painful is what they are.'

We keep going. My legs sliding back and forth, back and forth, and my arms pushing and pulling, pushing and pulling, and I know everything will ache, but my body feels good. Almost powerful even.

And I don't want to, but I wonder what Grace would say if she could see me here on the water. Ignoring for a moment the fact that I'm with a boy – a really, really nice but

I-must-not-fancy-him boy – and focusing instead on the fact that I'm moving, properly using my muscles in an exercising sort of way. She might faint, like, literally drop down on the riverbank. Cos I swear she's been telling me to do it for years. Not row – sorry, scull – exactly. But something.

'Our bodies are goddamn miracles!' she told me from a forearm stand a few months back. 'You need to love your body, Izzy.'

'I love McVitie's.'

'You can love both.'

I didn't mention how loving my body seemed impossible when I didn't even like it.

She'd be double thumbs up, I reckon. If she saw me now, I mean. But I can't do it, carry on thinking of her without bursting into a million tears, and today is a good day so I push all thoughts of her away and focus on my rhythm. Or complete lack of it.

'You're not bad!' Harry says.

I make this snuffly, snorty sound of disbelief, cos his voice is a nine-for-effort, three-for-actual-skill.

'Honestly,' he says, 'you've got potential.'

And I wonder if it could be true. Whether this body of mine could actually be OK at something.

'Let's hope you're right, otherwise you'll have been up at this ridiculous hour for nothing! What time do you have to be at college?'

'I don't,' Harry says, quick and maybe a little defensive. 'I don't go to college.'

'Sorry, I just assu—'

'What? That I wouldn't waste my fancy education and while my life away on the river?'

'Harry!' I let the blades rest in the water so I can turn to face him.

'Sorry.' Unlike that emoji-ish sad face of yesterday, today's is the real deal. 'Long story.'

'How long's the river?'

'It's actually the longest in the UK. People often make the mistake of thinking the Thames is the —'

'You know, I don't really care how long the river is, Harry. I was just suggesting you tell me that long story of yours.'

'It's honestly not that interesting.'

'And the debate around the UK's longest river is?!'

'I like you, Izzy,' he says. 'You say it how it is.'

I don't correct him because, if I'm honest, which Harry totally thinks I am, him believing I'm tough and straight-talking feels as good as Harry thinking my body has potential as a sculler.

'So…'

'What?' He manoeuvres the boat towards the bank, where he holds us in place as we bob up and down on the water.

'Why so touchy?'

'I'm a dropout.' Harry's voice is a week-old balloon some-one's forgotten to untie from a tree after a party.

'What do you mean?'

'I quit my A levels last year. Mum's still not over it. You don't go to *that* school –' he points up the hill to this huge red-brick building with its own clock tower – 'or your parents don't send you to *that* school, don't spend *all that money,*

164

Harry, all those thousands of pounds, Harry on *that* school for you to then tell them there are more important things in life than Greek and the Hunt!'

'You went hunting? At school? My god, how posh *are* you exactly?! Did you catch your own dinner – or supper? I bet you called it supper there, right?'

'We didn't hunt, not that kind of hunt anyway. But yes, we called the food we ate in the evening supper.'

'Ha! So pretty posh then.'

'The Hunt's actually cross-country running.'

'Ugh. I might literally prefer to go actual hunting and shoot a fox than go cross-country running through the woods!'

'It's not so bad really.'

'I'm kidding about the fox, right?!'

'I liked most of it really, but I didn't *love* it.'

'I love foxes.'

'And I thought, *What's the point, you know, in Mum and Dad spending all that money if I don't love it?*'

'Some of my best friends are foxes.'

Harry looks at me like, *I'm trying to be serious here.*

'Sorry, I *am* listening. I just didn't want you thinking I'm some kind of crazy fox killer. I would never kill a fox, not even to get out of cross-country!'

'OK, fox-lover, thanks for the clarification.'

'Sorry. Go on.'

'So after the first term of A levels, I told them I wasn't going back.'

'Did they freak out?'

'Well, if you count throwing my lacrosse stick on the fire freaking out, then yeah, they freaked out.'

'Hold on a minute? They threw your what on the fire?'

'My lacrosse stick.'

'Bloody hell, Harry. Like, seriously, how did you cope? I'm not sure what I'd do without my lacrosse stick.'

'Funny.'

'Sorry.'

''S all right,' he says, smiling properly. 'Dad pulled it out before too much damage was done.'

'Thank god. You had me worried then. A boy without his lacrosse stick doesn't bear thinking about.'

'I know, right!'

'And what about your mum and dad – are they recovering as well as the lacrosse stick?'

'Who knows?' He pushes us away from the bank and nods at the boat like I should crack on with my training. 'They're not exactly proud telling their mates I'm gonna be an apprentice, but they're no longer setting my possessions on fire.'

'An apprentice?'

'Painting and decorating.' He pauses then, like he's waiting for me to make a joke of it.

'Cool.'

'It is actually. Or it will be. I'm labouring at the moment. Got to wait till September for the apprenticeship. Mum's hoping I'll change my mind by then, go to uni or something. She doesn't get it at all, thought her clever little boy was going to grow up saving people's lives in a hospital, not stocking up on Dulux at B&Q.'

Harry pushes us away from the bank, gives me a nod to turn back into position and get my arms moving.

'What do you like about it? The painting, I mean.'

'The change. How in the space of a few days a place can go from looking and feeling a total mess to somewhere that's the opposite of that. To know I've helped make it happen. Stupid, right?'

'Not at all. Sounds great.' *Sounds familiar.*

It occurs to me I haven't thought about the blades and when to twist them, when to drop them into the water – I've just done it. For a few seconds at least, my body didn't feel awkward – it just worked.

'It's all very *Desert Island Discs* by the way,' I say.

'What?'

'*Desert Island Discs*. It's a radio programme. You'd love it. It's like your playlists. The guests have to pick eight songs to soundtrack their life. So you learn about their favourite music but through that you learn about the people too. And the best guests are the mavericks. Like you! You know, quitting your A levels, abandoning what was expected of you and finding something totally different that you love.'

'You reckon?'

'God, yeah! Those mavericks are the reason I listen! Even if they're already set up for massive success, they haven't been scared to screw it and have a go at something they think will bring them more joy.'

'So I'm a maverick?'

'Sounds better than dropout.'

'I'll tell my mum.'

'You totally should. And you should total—'

'Oh crap. You got something I can tell my boss to get him off my back too? I'm gonna be late. Put some sweat into it, Izzy. I've got to go.'

We make it back. Dry. Smiling. Looking forward to tomorrow at six A.M.

THIRTY-FOUR

I'm sure someone told me it takes twenty-one days to form a new habit, but Daniel had his nailed from the start. A photo every day since Mum and I scarpered. Thirteen of them so far. Unlucky for some, right? Thirteen reminders that he has my Jar of Sunshine. Thirteen reminders that he's stolen my light.

And yet.

There's enough to keep me from tumbling into his dark, because in the eight days since meeting Harry, other habits have been forming too. We're on the river each morning – just me, a boy and a boat – edging the meeting time earlier and earlier to stretch our one hour into two. But when we've reached the *see you later*s, the *tomorrow then*s and the only awkward moment of our mornings together – the will-we, won't-we, maybe, not-right-now possibility of A Kiss – those two hours still feel too short; I'd happily be here all day.

It's not just Harry – though believe me, he *is* pretty awesome – it's the river too. My body feels different here, as if the lumbering landlubber Izzy Chambers sheds her skin on the jetty and becomes something new, something else, something that's not just carried along by the river but works with it or against it upstream.

I once heard someone say, on the radio maybe, that there's an upside of moving far from home, that each time you go somewhere new you can leave something behind and become more of something else. I think about the old Izzy, the one from just two weeks ago, and she feels like one of those memories from when you're a tiny kid, like when I sat on a beach that was sand not Whitstable stone during a weekend in Norfolk, bucket for a hat, seaweed for knickers, and tipped my full packet of Wotsits upside down, filling the empty bag with sand before shovelling it into my mouth like I'd discovered some kind of delicacy. Mum tells the story and has the photo to prove it. But I can't feel it, how the grit would have wedged in my teeth, or clumped with Wotsit dust to turn my tongue a cheesy orange rough. So I look at the picture and it's sort of me but only because Mum tells me it is. I don't feel like I'm that girl in the photo.

Couple-of-weeks-ago Izzy is like years-and-years-ago Izzy. Like I can imagine everything that's happened to her, but she's not quite the Izzy of now. And so when Harry asks about me, what I like, what I'll study at uni, where in the world I'd most like to be, I'm not really sure. The answers are in there somewhere but they're groggy, like I've literally just woken up. Like I need a bit of time to adjust to the bright lights of the morning.

'You're looking stronger already,' Harry said yesterday, and he meant with the rowing, but when I told him I felt it, that change in my strength, *I* meant all over and all the way through. My arms, my legs, they seem more a part of me, which sounds stupid, right, but when I think about that bathroom with Jacob, that bedroom with Jacob, those moments all over with Daniel, there's this numbness to everything, like it's all been pushed to the back of somewhere, sat on maybe. But all this water and all this rowing, they wash and shake the pins and needles from me, get my blood rushing almost as much as the thought of that first-kiss list Harry's told me he's compiling. Thing is, he only ever mentions it when we're in the boat, when my back's to him, when logistically there's little chance of playing music or kissing lips. Not without falling in the river at least, and there wouldn't be much grace in that. That said, there's not much Grace in anything these days.

I miss her.

And I've thought about calling her. Cos, seriously, if Mum's bald head taught me anything it's screw it and try. What's the worst that can happen? Thing is, Grace is brilliant, amazing, ridiculously cool and that's why she's been such a brilliant, amazing, ridiculously cool stabiliser. And I've needed that, wanted that – couldn't have coped without that propping. But, for the first time in god knows how long, I feel like my own two feet can take my weight, like maybe I'm discovering something significant here.

I'm hoping it's not forever, this silence between us, that sometime soon I can phone Grace and tell her I'm sorry. I'm sorry for not being there when she needed cover, I'm sorry for shrinking not only from Daniel but from her too. For not telling her the truth about Daniel and Mum and me and all those different types of hurt he weaved around us. Sometime soon, I think, but not today, because today is a Jar of Sunshine day, the kind of day I'd like to bottle or bead on a string and wear close to my heart so I might feel its warmth on the days that aren't so bright.

Today is a day when, by 6.00 A.M., nothing and everything has happened. Because today is the day I'm standing on the bridge, definitely looking and definitely waiting and definitely feeling like the sky is within my reach. Like I have a place in it. Like my no-longer-landlubbery body can make its mark and not the kind of mark Daniel joked about when my 'planetary-sized bum left a crater in the sofa'.

Today is the day I become more of something else. And it doesn't matter that I don't know what that something else is, just that I feel it. I feel something in my bones and my flesh which isn't dread or revulsion. It's good.

'You're all right, Izzy Grace Chambers,' I say to my sort-of reflection in the river below, a reflection that's just a basic shape of me, no defining features. She could be anything, anyone, whatever she wants to be. It's nice to see her, to tell her she's doing OK, to not be staring into a mirror whispering how much I hate her, how stupid she is, how ugly, how all of everything that's happened is down to her. 'You're more than all right,' I say, eyes to the water then eyes to the sky. 'You might look like water but you, Izzy Grace Chambers, are tough!'

'You're also a bit bloody mental!'

Harry! His voice is a smile and it's a spark too.

'Sorry not sorry,' I say, turning to face him, to ask him, because I am Izzy Grace Chambers and I am bold, 'Would you mind if I kiss you, Harry?'

'No,' he says, and my heart tumbles into the river. 'No, I don't mind, I mean.'

And my heart leaps back up again, like salmon, as we walk closer and closer until everything meets, and he is Harry like Styles and I am Izzy Grace Chambers and together we are strength and sunshine and smiles and salmon hearts somersaulting on the river Severn.

And in this one moment everything is fucking perfect.

The sky is clear and blue above us.

I own it.

The sky is mine.

THIRTY-FIVE

'Time,' Harry calls as the alarm on his watch sounds seven thirty, when our limbs are done with the rowing and our mouths should really be but can't quite be done with the kissing.

I pull him back down to the jetty as he makes to gather his things.

'I've got to go, Iz.' He holds his calloused hands up as evidence. 'I'll walk you back home first though, yeah?'

'Really? Why the sudden chivalry?'

'Why the sudden kiss?'

'Touché, Harry!' I lean in for another one, then two.

'I'd do this all day if I could, but work calls.' He kisses me again. 'I've…' And again. 'Got…' And again. 'To…' And again. 'Go.'

'Sorry.' I pull back, and I mean I'm sorry for the kisses delaying him but also for those white lies I've told when he's asked about why I'm in Shropshire. Mum's been pretty ill, I've told him. We've come on holiday to celebrate her being well. My dad is dead, and it's just the two of us. I haven't mentioned that the illness is Daniel and the hotel's a safe house for abused women and kids.

'How about I walk you to work instead?' I say, wishing I could dive into the water to tame my reddening cheeks, swim all the way back to the refuge, maybe, so there's no chance of

Harry discovering the real reasons I came to this town. 'Save you being late.' And though I'm smiling, I wonder if he hears it, how I'm porcelain now, a tall vase brushed by the untruths swirling around me, wobbling, threatening to crack.

'If you're sure,' Harry says, his hand still in its kissing position on my jaw and below my chin, same place Daniel would hold Mum when he was sorry, so sorry, and Mum would nod into his fingers, and I crossed mine, as I stood just outside the door of their 'disagreements', hoping that maybe this time his apology was true.

I put my hand over Harry's now and hold it there, absorbing its tenderness, willing him to trust in me, this new Izzy who's as much a novice in romance as she is in a boat.

'So, tomorrow's Saturday,' he says.

'That fancy education obviously served you well, Harry.'

'Ha ha!' He nudges me with his elbow, pulls me back in. 'No labouring! We could have a whole day.'

'On the river?'

'I was thinking we take our relationship to the next level.'

And despite all the efforts of pushing those experiences of weeks-ago-Izzy into the ground, maybe I stiffen.

'Land, Izzy! I was thinking we could do something on land. And not *that* kind of something! What kind of man do you take me for?'

I think of all the other kinds of men and don't say a word.

'What do you reckon?'

'I'll need to check my diary.'

Harry looks at me, like, *really?*

I make this whole show of pulling my phone from my

pocket and looking at Saturday 24 June. 'It's tricky, see, cos I have this very important meeting at nine and a very important lunch at twelve and a very impor—'

But over the calendar comes notification of a WhatsApp from Jacob, and from the way my heart's lurching, tomorrow might be irrelevant because tomorrow might never come.

'A very important what, Izzy?' And Harry, Harry with his beautiful big smile, he's reaching over, playfully grabbing my phone to check out 'what could possibly be more important than this'. He kisses me, waving the phone behind his back just of my reach and, thank god, just out of his sight. 'You're so incredible, Izzy,' he mumbles into my lips. 'It's untrue.'

Maybe it is. Untrue, I mean. And Harry will know as soon as he stops kissing me and looks at my phone and sees what Jacob has to say.

Tick tock, Fingers. My place. Tomorrow. Go down on me or go down in history. Here's a little reminder of what's at stake.

If I hadn't opened the message, the words and photo would have remained hidden behind the empty calendar I could have filled with hours and hours of Harry. But now, if Harry so much as glances at the screen, he'll see it in all its glory: the dirty real me.

'I'm sorry, Harry,' I say, pulling away from the kiss, snatching the phone before he sees the truth in it.

He looks at me, like, *I don't get it*, and I know he never will.

'I can't do this,' I tell him. 'Not with you.' And though I mean it like, *you're too good*, it comes out like, *you're not good enough*.

I hear it, the plummet of his heart when it drops into the river, as I run faster and faster, never outrunning the shame.

THIRTY-SIX

I'm as bad as Mum. With that hope of hers, I mean. That stupid hope that silence was the best tactic. That keeping quiet would push the worst things to arm's length until better things could push them further and further away.

I've tried calling. I need to talk to you, Izzy. About Jacob.

Call me back.

Please.

I don't want to talk about Jacob. Not to Max. Because what exactly can he tell me that I don't already know?

I've barely thought about it, what Jacob did. What I let him do. How I lay there and gave him everything and nothing in one. Sure, the weight of him has pressed down on me at night sometimes. Shower water has felt like his wet breath on my neck. And all that Intensive Repair used not just as conditioner but kind of desperately as body wash too – even that has failed to rid my skin of his touch. It sounds so gentle, right? Touch. And Jacob wasn't gentle so maybe he didn't just touch me. So what *is* the word then, for what he did?

Yeah, I've barely thought about it. But it's been there, I s'pose, same way an owner's smell can stick around in their house once they're gone. I remember how the flat we had stank of nothing specific but everything that wasn't us. The walls. The carpets. The air even. Months of vacuuming and plug-in air fresheners, but it was still there, weaving into our clothes and our hair until either we got rid of it or maybe we just smelt of it too.

I smell of Jacob. Every second his dirty hands were on me has me stinking of what we did between those Monster Munched sheets of his.

I've been waiting for Harry to spot it when he's kissed me. Waiting for him to taste it. Whatever sense is strongest, it would have found me out eventually. But I kept kissing him anyway, that genetic false hope of mine willing the bad stuff to sail away down the river so I might get on with the good.

But it doesn't leave you. Even when your head tries to silence it, it's still there. Like Jacob and his threats and his photos. It's all still there.

Maybe I need another jar. The opposite of a Jar of Sunshine. Maybe I need to whisper all these things I can't say into a jar and put a lid on it. Seal it tight. Pandora's box in reverse.

I wonder what Daniel's doing with it now, my Jar of Sunshine, where he puts it when he's not taking those photos. There's another one when I double-, triple-, quadruple-check that WhatsApp from Jacob: my jar, perched on the mantel-piece in the sitting room between a picture of Daniel and a picture of my dad.

I need it here. Because listening to danandcharlie95 is nowhere near enough to warm all this cold and sullied blood charging through me as I run to the refuge, to Mum.

She's at the window when I come up the front path, pressed to it almost, the sadness and seriousness of her face exagger-ated by that bald head she's run over each day with a razor, her eyes as sharp as the blade, and her voice, when she looks up and tra-la-las a good morning, as smooth as her skin when she was first done. The bald made her bold, but *this* morning, not yet shaved, there's a fuzziness that extends beyond her scalp, softening the backbone she's held so rigid in the last few days.

'We need to talk,' she says.

My phone beeps with another photo from Daniel: that framed picture of my dad I kept on a shelf inside my wardrobe is now smashed to pieces on the floor.

And Mum's right: we do need to talk. I need to tell her about Harry and Jacob and how my heart is drowning in the river. I need to tell her about Daniel and all my broken sunshine he's threatening to destroy, but Mum's already starting.

'Izzy,' she says, as she takes me by the hand towards our bedroom, straight past the kitchen, where Ava, spoon clattering into her Weetabix bowl when she sees me, comes running out in her summer school dress, hands raised and already singing.

But Kate's straight on the case, scooping Ava up and away, eyeballing Mum, like, *you can do this*. And I look at Kate, like, *what?*, but she just smiles, like, *everything's fine*, and their glances feel like a conspiracy.

'That appointment,' Mum says, when we're still in the hallway, eyes fixed on our bedroom door, which she closes behind us before sitting me down on the bed, our necks cricked because of the top bunk, which looks like it's literally pressing this huge weight upon her shoulders.

'For your hair?' And I want to yell that her bald head is nothing compared to my broken soul.

'My hair?'

'Yeah, your hair appointment!' I say, like we have all this time to waste. 'The one you went to with Kate instead of me, probably because you thought *I* would try to talk you out of *this*.' I point at her head.

'Oh no,' she says, 'a hairdresser didn't do this. Kate did.'

For some reason this adds to all the hurt, not a big gut punch or anything, but a paper-cut kind of hurt, as I imagine the two of them prepping and giggling, gasping as the first strands of hair dropped to the floor. Grace and I would spend hours braiding, on our beds, on the sofa, on the bus even, fingers constantly pulling and coaxing, then soothing and smoothing when the pulling and coaxing was too much. Even when it hurt, there was a happiness in our intimacy, in the physicality of our friendship, in how Grace was the only one with whom my body could properly flump down on to a bed, let it all hang out and breathe.

The paper-cut pain spreads into my middle, where Grace runs right through me in name only these days, and I sink into the bed, fighting back the tears I've been fighting back since Jacob's message. Since way before that maybe.

'The appointment,' Mum says, the repetition quite clearly a delaying tactic. 'The appointment,' she starts over, 'was at a clinic.'

And she must think I know exactly what that means because her eyes are on me, like, *say something*, but I just shrug, like, *yeah?*

And my mum, she takes this breath, and in this voice that sounds like my mother's but can't possibly be my mother's, because my mother wouldn't be saying these words, she tells me, 'Izzy, I'm having an abortion.'

And there's the big gut punch right there.

'You're what?'

'I'm having an abortion,' she says, not even stumbling over the A word, just putting it out there like she's having a jacket potato for lunch. 'Don't look at me like that, Izzy,' she says, but there's nothing I'm doing that I'm doing on purpose – not my silence, not my rolling dollopy tears, not that paper cut that's split me open from the top of my chest to my pelvis – so all those gut reactions spill out of me, spewing on to my mother, who's statue still, and the gut reaction scoffs at the irony of it, how she can appear so lifeless when there's so much life inside her. For now.

And I don't get it, because she's always insisted it was never an option. That she never even considered it. 'You were a keeper,' she said, those few times I asked her, but then I think of everything I've tried to hide from Harry, for my own sake as much as his, and I wonder if Mum was also trying to hide the parts of her she wasn't so proud of, to build herself up as this better version of herself who would never have thought of getting rid of her child. But she must have done. Thought of it, I mean. If she's thinking of it now she must have thought of it then. When I was inside her and she had the choice to say yes or no.

'Is that what you wish you'd had with m—'

'Izzy,' she says, but I'm sick of it, my name in her mouth like it doesn't constantly taste of regret. 'It was different with you.'

'It was worse, you mean. You were sixteen. You're thirty-three now, Mum. More grown-up. More capable. More motherly even? Or not, it seems.' And, even before the words are fully formed, I'm pretty sure Mum can't deal with this. 'Makes sense, I suppose.' I lean in so close I can see her pulse quickening in her neck. 'Not exactly mother of the year, are you?'

'Please,' she says, but I'm not sure what she's pleading for. 'I'd change it all if I could.'

'I bet you would.' Because without me she would never have been in Whitstable, she would never have met Daniel, she would never have been sitting with a bald head in a women's refuge talking about aborting another baby she doesn't want.

'Not that, Izzy. Not you. I'd never change *you*.'

But she's too slow to catch me as I run from the room, from the refuge, from everything that's ever happened because I was born.

You should have seen my dad's face when he first saw me, when Mum and I turned the corner into the park, and he rose from the bench where he'd been sitting with his guitar in a case beside him. I've seen reunions on TV, when long-lost relatives appear to move in slow motion, unsure how to greet this person who, if things had been different, could have been a stabiliser during their wobblier moments in life. Dad wasn't slow mo. He moved so fast I asked Mum later when he popped to the loo if he was related to Dash from *The Incredibles*. 'No, love,' she said, voice like a bunch of balloons sky high with helium. 'He just couldn't wait a second longer to meet you.'

He wanted me, no doubt about that. His hug, his song, his necklace. I was his sunshine. My birth may have caused all sorts of darkness for my mother, but in that moment, for my father, I was a pure blast of light.

All of these photos, all of these images – Daniel, Jacob, Dad – thrash with each step, faster and faster like a strobe, until I reach the ticket machine, rummaging through Mum's purse, which I grabbed from the side as I left, tapping in her PIN number and whispering to Dad how sorry I am for ever letting him go.

I'm getting that Jar of Sunshine back.

I won't let Daniel have it.

It's mine.

THIRTY-SEVEN

The train doesn't feel as good as I expected. When I was running, my feet couldn't move quickly enough. Same for my thoughts, my plan. Hah! That's a joke, right? Because when I bolted all I really knew was that I needed to get to my Jar of Sunshine before Daniel did something too permanent. So other than stealing Mum's purse and getting to Whitstable, there is no plan. There's just this stupid girl who's got to take three different trains and wait more than four hours before she even gets within walking distance of a strawberry jam jar filled with yellow beads. And that's assuming it's still there, still in one piece. When you put it like that…

Only it's not like that, is it? Because it's not just a jam jar and they're not just beads.

Along with their eight pieces of music, the *Desert Island* castaways are permitted a luxury. No practical items allowed, and that's fine with me, because if I were stranded, what I'd want most from my luxury is hope. That's why I ran. Because it was doing something other than accepting my fate. Because it was remembering my dad and how he'd wanted me to keep the sunshine close to my heart. Because it was believing that if I can just get the jar from Daniel then maybe I won't be quite so lost in the dark.

But the train doesn't feel as good as I expected.

I always thought I preferred to face the direction of travel, but when I switch seats so I can't see where I'm going, it feels something like the river with Harry and —

Do not think of Harry.

Harry.

Do not think of Harry.

Harry.

Do not think of Harry.

Harry.

Music. I need music. A distraction from the do-not-think-of-Harry/thinking-of-Harry rut I'm in. Harry would suggest a runaway playlist, but obviously I'm not thinking of Harry so I can't do a runaway list because that will just carry me back to him.

Do not think of Harry.

Harry.

Music, Izzy.

Harry.

Goddamn it.

I swipe away two, three, four missed calls from Mum as Spotify suggests I jump back into my Top Listens from the last few months, and right there at the pinnacle of my most-played tracks is a song from Pink's *Greatest Hits…So Far!!!* It's there thanks to Grace. See, it's not only Harry who has play-lists. Grace has them too, only she's not so prescriptive. Because it's not like she said, 'Here, Izzy, you *must* listen to Pink, track eighteen. It's number one on this *self-esteem* list I've made you.' What Grace *did* do, on the first day at college after *that* party, when Jacob used the three-fingers-or-four photo to make me fair game for general abuse, was insist I go back to hers for a Pot Noodle dinner and a bed mosh, which basically means we jumped furiously up and down on her mattress to a load of music I now realise she'd probably preselected to maximise my chances of sweating out the shame.

'*Woah, woah, woah! Here!* On the bed! Now! You are *not* stopping there, babe.' She pulled me back up with both arms, refusing to let go even when I relented and began to leap as told. 'This song,' she said, pausing the jumps so she could clutch my hands to her chest. 'This song is *you*, Izzy. This song is *us*,' she said, and 'Fuckin' Perfect' blasted hard from her phone. Clearly the song wasn't a cure. It was a help though. Our hearts pumped not just blood but mutual adoration to our riotous and fuckin' perfect limbs.

Cos that's the power of music, right? It can wrap itself around you like a big noisy duvet, a thick wad of feathery comfort that protects you from the outside world, muffling all those other words you don't want to hear. Even when you're not literally playing it, you can run through the lyrics in your head and the power of them gets into your bloodstream, makes you feel for a moment like you're as kick-ass as Pink, who has no problem telling the world to do one when it doesn't play fair.

So yeah, I sit with my back in the direction of travel, ignoring another four, five calls from Mum to play it over and over. Not just the song but that night. How Grace wouldn't let me leave until she'd styled my hair, painted my nails and made me laugh so hard I nearly peed my pants. And how I'd sulked a bit when I'd come back from the loo to find her curled into her pillow, whispering into her phone and twirling her curls like some cliché who'd rather be with her girlfriend than stuck with the college joke. 'Gotta go. You too,' she said to Nell. I knelt down, rummaging through my rucksack so she wouldn't see how my face crumpled at the sound of their love. And I'd thought then that Grace had only brought me home, fed me dirty noodles and danced my heart out because there'd been nothing better on offer. Second choice. But I wonder now whether she actually put me first. Cancelled her plans with Nell to be with me. And I'm not saying that after the whole Jacob thing Grace was fuckin' perfect, but maybe she was closer to fuckin' perfect than I thought.

I read her email over and over as we speed towards Kent, and while the anger's obvious, it's the underlying disappointment that gets me most. *You're supposed to be my best friend*, she wrote, and I think of all the times she more than lived up to her responsibilities as mine. Cos the thing is, maybe Grace didn't really understand about Daniel, but she stepped up anyway, like that sixth sense she claimed we had was a literal thing, like even if she didn't know what pushed me, if she ever saw me wobbling, she sure as hell wasn't going to stand back and watch me fall.

Until now.

Because surely she must've been wondering where I've been the last few weeks. However extreme her fury, if they *are* real, Grace's inklings should be twitching enough for her to screw the fact she asked me to leave her alone for a bit and to come find me, or at least send another, kinder email, or just a text maybe – a *You OK?* would do. But there's been nothing. So maybe, like Mum, Grace has realised a life without me would be so much less stressful, so much more fun.

But I miss her. I miss her so hard my danced-out heart's totally gutted, and my riotous and fuckin' perfect limbs sit as pathetic and immobile as the goddamn crisp packet someone's tossed on the train's filthy floor.

THIRTY-EIGHT

Next stop Whitstable, and there's this literal tug at my heart, pulling it back into my chest where it melds into the rest of me, and for a few seconds at least, there's a physical relief that, no matter the shit fest of my problems, I'm almost home. Thing is, there's no way it can last, cos it's not home, is it? Nowhere is, I tell myself, wishing when I get off the train that the air didn't smell so much like my childhood.

It's proper hot, and as they leave the station, two commuters stop to roll up their sleeves, that Friday feeling in the smiles they share with each other, how they nod before heading their separate ways to their normal families and their normal weekends by the sea. One heads down the road towards Daniel's house, so it's not like I'm actually following him, not really, cos I'd be heading that direction anyway. He's about the same age as Mum, and I wonder if she had met him instead of Daniel, whether she would have kissed him, gone to Paris with him, moved us in with him, married him, kept her job and her strength and a baby if they'd made one.

When he struggles with his bag and his jacket and the key in the lock, a woman appears, toddler at her knee, kiss on his lips and they're gone, behind closed doors where no one knows what happens, right? But it has to be better than what happened behind ours. If you'd have peeked through our letterbox, the first thing you'd have seen would have been *happiness*, but that was just the hallway. I think we all know everywhere else was anything but.

I sit on the low carpark wall, doing my best to avoid looking like some weirdo stalker, long enough for the door to open and the three of them to emerge, the man my mum didn't meet or kiss or marry now changed into beach clothes, into Dad mode, holding the kid's hands then lifting her onto his shoulders as his partner looks on, laughing at the dribble snaking its way down her daughter's chin and onto the hair of the man my mum didn't meet or kiss or marry. I literally can't move until they've gone.

My dad would have been like that, I think. That smile, remember, when he first saw me, just a few hundred metres from here in the park where he stood up from the bench, which is still there when I abandon the route to Daniel's house and walk instead towards the memory of my dad, which is tracing paper, too thin and too transparent to make a ghost of him even. Because I didn't have enough time to grasp the bulk of him, to memorise his walk, his mannerisms, his voice. It'd be sunshine though, right? A big yellow declaration that abortion had never been an option, and unlike Mum's, it'd be true. *But only* – says a voice, small but mean, in my head – *because he didn't know, did he? He didn't know about you until it was too late, until you were already here, holding your mother's hand, holding your mother back, a five-year-old weight around your mother's neck.*

What if she'd told him when she first found out she was pregnant? Because he was just seventeen then, with his whole life stretching out ahead of him, and – how could I not have realised this before? – that life would have stretched even further if it weren't for me and his obligation to visit. If I hadn't been born, he wouldn't have needed to come to Whitstable. He'd have been far away from that motorway and the lady with her attention on her mobile instead of the road. His car wouldn't have flipped over into the bank. He wouldn't have been cut free by firemen, already dead, meaning that the choice he made to have me in his life was the choice that killed him.

So no wonder Mum won't risk it again, because that first choice *she* made was a domino and everything that came after fell down.

'Fingers!'

I hear him before I see him, but there's no doubt it's Jacob Mansfield behind me, his voice a whole bunch of entitlement and scorn.

'Come to give evidence, have you?'

When I turn around, Jacob's sneering, like all he sees is the photograph of me on his monument bed.

And then he's on the bench next to me, his hands on my shoulders, no actual force, but my panic's a coat made of lead, pushing me down, further and further from the sky.

'Or maybe you've realised you want some after all.' He slides closer until there's no space between us. 'Give us a kiss then, Izzy.'

The lead coat grows a lead hat and lead boots and I'm

totally going nowhere as Jacob leans in, face like a catapult about to fling its worst.

'Thought it'd make me go away, did you?' His hand's on the exact same part of my chin as Harry's was this morning. It's only the pressure that's different, but it changes everything. 'Be a good girl then – tell me why you grassed me up.' He squeezes and everything changes again.

'Leave me alone, Jacob.' And I'd swear the words are only in my head, but the look on his face says otherwise, their volume increasing the tension on that catapult so Jacob's suddenly right up on me, nose to nose, mouth to mouth, voice as dark and underground as a well.

'Leave me alone, Jacob,' he repeats back to me, his impression making me sound squeaky, pathetic, weak.

Rising to his feet, he bends over me, stealing every inch of my sky. One hand grasps at my shoulder, his forehead pushing against mine as his other hand pinches at the fat that folds over my jeans. But it's all just a different kind of pressure, the tugging and the pulling. No pain. Just drowsiness and surrender. The simplicity of it so familiar I let myself drift. Because this is what happens to girls like me with boys like Jacob. This is what we deserve. And I fall deeper and deeper into the well, away from the sun and the moon, where the embers of that tough, don't-take-any-shit Izzy are immediately starved of air.

'Why'd you tell the college about our deal, Izzy?'

Jacob's voice is a yank into the now, and I stare right at him, no clue what he means but sure at least of what he'll do to me.

'Eh?'

'I didn't. I don't know what yo—'

'You didn't? Really? Why was I pulled into the head's office at lunchtime then? Admit it. You told them.'

'I swear I —'

'I swear I —' Jacob mimics. And it's his copycatting that does it. Something about it is the same old, same old story. Like those boys on the river and how they're all caught up in this just being the way of things. This assumption that they'll shut me down.

'You swear what, Izzy?'

'I didn't tell college,' I say. Hard. Clear. Aloud.

'No?' Jacob doesn't break the eye lock he has on me. 'Well, who did then?'

'Steph,' says a voice from somewhere behind. 'Steph told them.'

'Grace?' Just her name in my mouth is a shot of grit to my gut. I pull myself away from Jacob's grasp.

'Steph?' He's looking from me to Grace, like, *what the actual?* 'Who the fuck is Steph?'

'My *mum* knows about this?'

'I'm sorry, Iz.' Grace is all out of breath from appearing out of nowhere. 'But when Max called me this morning and told me what's been go—'

'Max? You fucking what?' Jacob is bigger suddenly, chest puffed not with air but all this raging bad blood.

'Max told *me. I* told Izzy's mum. Izzy's mum told *college*. It's *really* not that complicated. Even for a *Neanderthal* brain like yours, Jacob.'

Grace comes over, takes my hand as she sits down next to

me, totally not intimidated by the extra height she's granting Jacob, just giving off this air, like, *we're not playing this game any more*.

'Fuck off, Jacob,' she says.

And, yeah, maybe there are more eloquent ways to end it but 'fuck off' is so fuckin' perfect for this moment that it'll do.

THIRTY-NINE

'I've missed you,' I say, kind of breathless, like we're in a love scene, which I guess we sort of are.

'You too.' She's pulling me into a hug already.

'I'm sorry.'

'I'm sorry.'

And we're five again.

'Jinx!'

'Jinx!'

Pinky-linking our fingers to make a wish.

We watch Jacob skulk off, hands in his pockets, kicking the odd stone, head still not hanging despite everything.

I'd assumed anyone else knowing about the photos would feel worse than this. I'd assumed I'd be mortified but, really, what I feel most is relieved. Like that power has actually shifted. Like it'll no longer be so easy for Jacob, for anyone, to steal my sky. Oh, but my mum though!

'God, did you really have to tell my mum? My *mum*! Eugh.'

Grace must assume the roll of my eyes is at her, not at the thought of my mother, who probably thinks those photos are just further evidence of why she should never have had me.

'I'm *sorry*,' she says. 'I didn't know *what* to do.'

'And Mum did, did she?' Cos Mum's decision-making isn't exactly on point right now.

'Well, yeah. I mean, Jacob's *suspended* while they *investigate*, so that's something.'

'S'pose.'

When I've imagined my reunion with Grace, it's always been a bit more upbeat than the flat line I'm currently riding.

'C'mon,' she says, 'give me one of those Izzy *Grace* Chambers smiles.'

And I can't help it – no matter all that heartache I've left up in Shropshire, being with Grace again is enough to make me grin.

'There you *go*! See, *Grace* to the *rescue*!'

She's only joking, I know. And I get it, honestly I do, and I am grateful, totally one hundred percent grateful for her help, but just now, before her perfectly timed arrival, I was on the brink of something. The fluttering in my belly no longer felt so much like fear, but like the embers from the river were growing wings, turning into a phoenix maybe, figuring out its flight.

It's not that I don't love how Grace is here, holding me, propping me, because aside from the last few weeks, it's where she's always been, how we've always worked. Grace: the leader, the decision maker. Izzy: one step behind. But maybe I'm done with being the one at the back, awaiting rescue. Because sure, it's been fine letting Grace take the helm while I take her tail. But it was a lot less than fine when I trudged along, a similar but different kind of submission when Jacob was the one in charge, doing what he was doing while I said neither yes nor no cos little Izzy was too much at the back to be heard. And Daniel? A lot less than fine doesn't even begin to cover it; how he made himself the front man, not only pushing Mum and me to the rear but pushing us down too, leaving us sprawled on our backs, barely able to move.

'You know, I'm gonna try to do a bit of rescuing myself from now on. Girl power and all that!'

'Goddamn *right* you are,' Grace says, and in true love-scene style we fall into each other's arms, both of us swimming in a goddamn river of tears.

FORTY

'Hot choc?'

Before I even nod, Grace is already on it: Cadbury's, milk, spoon, whisk, two mugs and two chairs pulled out from the kitchen table so I can fess up, she says. '*Jesus*, Iz, this is some *serious* shit.'

'You first,' I tell her, because surely it wasn't actually some sixth sense that had her in the park at the same time as me and Jacob.

'Find My Friend,' she says.

I look at her, like, *genius*, remembering how the first thing we did when we got our phones was set them to see where the other was. And it'd been fun to start off with, checking in on Grace's whereabouts so I'd know when she was on her way. The novelty wore off pretty quickly though because, back then, there was never much distance between us, not for long anyway, but I'll admit, when she and Nell got together, I'd use it to get a better idea of what they were up to. Without me. You know, to see exactly how far away Nell was stealing my friend.

'How long did it take you to cave?'

Grace raises her eyebrows, like, *don't get too cocky*, but, sad as it is, I really do want to know.

'Honestly? About six hours after sending *that* email,' she

says, and our laughter's like the sound my Jar of Sunshine makes when I shake it, like thin streams of yellow elbowing their way through a cloud. 'It just seemed *really weird*, you know, that you and your mum would go off like that. And seriously, *Shropshire*? Like, yeah, if it were *Vegas*, I'd have been, like, *I get it*, but flippin' *Shrewsbury*? I'd never even heard of it. So I asked Daniel —'

'You did what?'

'I asked Daniel where you'd gone.'

My eyes must be spinning sirens or something, cos Grace is all 'No, no, no, I didn't tell him I'd been *tracking* you or anything. *God*, Izzy, I wouldn't want him thinking I'm some kind of *stalker*! I just asked him if he knew where you were staying, when you'd be back and all that. I promise I didn't give *anything* away.'

'Crap.' And my sirens are louder and brighter this time, not because of Grace, not directly anyway, but because if *she's* been able to keep an eye on me, maybe Daniel has too. And I remember that night Mum and I first arrived in the refuge, how Elizabeth had told us to change the settings on our phones, and I'd been so scared of missing something from Grace that I hadn't even thought about Daniel. 'I'm so stupid.'

'Er, *Pink* alert, *Pink* alert!' Grace says, teeing up her phone so she can sing about getting rid of all those negative voices in my head. 'You are *not* stupid, Izzy!' Her palms are pressed against my ears, rattling my skull. 'Now, repeat after me: *I*, Izzy Grace Chambers…' And her voice is a piss-take but her eyes are serious as hell.

'I, Izzy Grace Chambers…'

'*Am totally, absolutely, undeniably, literally, seriously, fuckin'* *perfect.*'

'Am totally? Absolutely?'

'*Undeniably, literally, seriously…*'

'Undeniably? Literally? Seriously?'

'*Fuckin' perfect.*'

'Fuckin' perfect.'

'Good. Now say it like you mean it, Izzy.'

'I, Izzy Grace Chambers, am totally, absolutely, undeniably, literally, seriously, fuckin' perfect.'

'Bravo.'

'As much as I appreciate the pep talk, Grace, I really am. Stupid, I mean.'

She slaps her hand against her forehead, like, *do I have to make you say this shit again?*

'I mean it. If Daniel's been able to track me…' And the life and death of things becomes clearer then, even to me, when I tell Grace about that time Daniel followed Mum to Canterbury, trailing the bus in his car and parking on double yellows so he didn't lose sight of her when she got off.

'Your deception's cost me seventy-five pounds in parking penalties, Stephanie. You do know, don't you, how difficult things have been financially since you decided to give up your job and be a lady of leisure?' Daniel crouched on the floor in front of her and, yeah, he may have been on his knees, but with his bared teeth, those lines between his eyes, how they made even his nose look like a weapon when he grimaced, you couldn't get any more opposite of bowing down. 'Where did you get the money for your bus fare?'

And because her answer was a low mumble, Daniel repeated it, eyes moving from her to me to be sure I was listening.

'Isabel's purse?' he said.

Mum, who even when he hit her usually stayed quiet and calm, was proper weeping then, big chokes in her throat, tears on her hands and staining her top. All that washable hurt no one else would ever see.

'Why'd you do it, Stephanie? Sneak around behind my back?'

'I didn't mean —'

'You didn't mean to *what*? Steal money from your daughter? Tell lies to your husband?'

And that's what made talking about it so impossible, because those words, Daniel's accusations, they don't sound the same when I say them cos, in the black and white of things, everything he was saying was kind of true.

'I'm sorry,' she said.

'And then you have the gall to ask why I can't trust you?'

It was always worse when he stopped shouting. That was when Mum would normally indicate I should leave, just a nod of her head or a twitch of her hand, but that day, she looked more the other way from me than ever, like the shame had been doubled, because of the cash she'd taken from my purse maybe.

But even if she had given me the sign to go, I would've stayed.

'I'm only going to ask you once, Stephanie. Who was he?'

'Luke,' Mum said.

Somehow she didn't even flinch when the tepid tea Daniel

was pouring from her cup over her head ran into her eyes and mouth.

'Luke now, is it?' And from his voice, it sounded like Luke had predecessors, but I swear Mum hadn't been out in, like, forever.

'He's my cousin.'

'You're fucking your cousin?' Daniel turned to me. 'You must be so proud, Isabel: it's not just theft your mother keeps in the family.'

I knew not to say anything. There were rules in these moments, and the three of us each knew them by heart.

'I'm not sleeping with him.' Her voice was pure monotone.

'I saw you kiss him.'

'On the cheek.'

'He paid for lunch, Stephanie. He will have wanted something in return.'

'He was being kind. I have no money, Daniel.' And though she wouldn't have meant for it to come through, we all heard it, that shard of accusation, just sharp enough to slice through the thin line between Daniel's buttoned-up threat and his hands-on fury.

You'd think you'd have to look away when your stepdad sucker-punches your mum in her belly, that if you were going to watch it, it would at least be through your fingers. But like Mum in the waterfall of tea, I barely even blinked.

I played my part, waited for it to be over, for Daniel to make his promises and for my heart to stop threatening to burst through my jumper and smother Daniel in hate.

Funny how people think love has sole possession of the heart. They're wrong, you know. Hate lives there too. I feel the deep throb of it now as I tell Grace about the wet patch that wasn't just Tetley that Mum left on the chair when she got up to go have the bath Daniel made such a show of running for her.

'With bubbles,' I say to Grace, 'and a candle. But all I could smell was the piss. I'm not even sure she knew she'd done it. Weed herself, I mean.' I picture Mum in the refuge this morning, summoning the guts to tell me about the abortion. 'Imagine being that scared.'

'Did you speak with her about it?'

'No. None of it.' I scramble at the buttons on my phone. 'He's dangerous, Grace. If he was that suspicious about Mum going out for lunch, imagine how he'll be now. Two weeks of us missing. Two weeks of his rage.' I turn off the location services on my phone. 'He'll have been looking for us. What if he's managed to use Find My Friend?' I check the settings. 'He was always reading Mum's emails and stuff – what if he had access to *my* phone as well as hers? He could have added himself as a friend, right?' I breathe only when I see it's Grace's name alone in my friend list.

'It's *OK*, Iz.' And my best friend's body is a blanket as she wraps herself around me, pulling me into her and stroking my hair.

'I've been so selfish. I knew what he was like, but I still —'

'It was a *mistake*. You've changed it now – he can't find you.'

But it's not the phone I'm talking about. It's the way I left things with Mum. The things I said. The judgements I made. The accusations I threw.

Far as I know, there's no button to fix any of that.

FORTY-ONE

'I can't *believe* it,' Grace says for, like, the tenth time in an hour. And the thing is, saying it out loud, all that abuse after abuse after abuse, neither can I. 'He's always so...so nice,' she says finally. She stretches her leg across the bed, prods my thigh with her toe, checking I'm really here maybe, that what I'm saying is really true. 'You know what I mean?'

And I do, yeah, because I remember the days before they were married when I wished Daniel was my stepdad, the days later when I was so happy he was, how they were all of the days in the beginning, some of the days in the middle, but none of the days in the end.

Because he wasn't a stepdad by then – he was a monster.

Daniel Chambers. A dad. An actual real-life dad. And though the thought of it lurches my heart like vomit into my mouth, the only other option does too.

'Mum's pregnant.' I try so hard to keep my opinion out of my voice.

'*Shiiiiiiiiiit!* She's not *keeping* it though, is she?' And it seems so easy, the way Grace puts it, like it's some done deal, not even calling 'it' a baby, like getting rid of 'it' is the only way.

'No.' And, though it's only two letters, Grace, with her sixth sense and all that, obviously picks up on something more than just the tiny word.

'What? Izzy?' she says, and there's a judgement in *her* tone too, like, *surely you can't expect her to have 'it'?*

But I do. I know it's all sorts of awful, but I do.

'Seriously?' And her face, it's how I imagine it was when she was writing that email, a tattoo of disappointment in her frown. 'You want her tied to that man for the *rest* of her life?'

'She wouldn't have to be.' I jump in cos I've already thought this through. 'I'd help her, Grace. Mum did it all on her own when I was born, but this time, she'd have *me*. I'd take care of the baby. *And* her.'

But where there was disappointment, there's disbelief.

'Did you actually hear everything you've just told me, Izzy? Everything Daniel's done to your mum? How calculated he's been? How vicious?' I can't even look to see what's scrawled across her face now, but her voice is a big warning bell of a clue, as Grace pitches everything as a question, not because she doesn't believe what I've told her but because she clearly can't believe I don't see it as a reason, a justification, for Mum's decision. 'I mean, bloody hell, Iz, are you *actually* saying you don't believe in a *woman's right to choose?*'

'You sound like one of your feminist leaflets.'

'And *you* sound like a *nob*. For fuck's sake, Izzy, even in the most *normal* of circumstances, your mum shouldn't have to have a baby if she doesn't want to, but *this*! Are you *seriously* telling me you think she should have a child she doesn't want, a child that belongs to a man who, from what you've said, has *manipulated* her, *beaten* her, made her *leave* everything she knows to live in a safe house because she thinks if she stays with him she might *actually* die? Is that what you *really* think, Izzy?'

And she's off the bed, pacing the room, biting the skin around the edges of her fingernails, shaking her head like what I've said is on the same level of wicked as Daniel.

I wish I could put Mum's secret back in its box, but it's out there now, and though I'd rather not talk about it any more, Grace is eyeballing me for an answer.

'She managed with me.' It's all I can come up with and Grace obviously isn't having any of it, cos she stops still right in front of me, stares like she's not budging until I have the guts to at least look her in the face.

But when I catch her gaze, she shifts from that wild outrage to a quiet kind of wisdom. 'Yeah, the difference is, Iz, the only issue with your dad was that he was a teenager. Daniel's a psychopath. It's not the same.'

And I get it. I get that Mum loved my dad. That my dad loved my mum. That the love between them was normal, genuine. Not soaked with fear. I get all of that, honestly, I do, but Mum kept *me* a secret. She could do the same again. 'Daniel wouldn't have to know.'

'I don't even know if that's *legal*, and even if it is, don't you think he'd *find out*? *Hunt* your mum down? And then what would happen? To your *mum*? To the *baby*? To *you*? You're not making any sense, Iz.'

And maybe I'm not, but it's clear to me. 'She's my mum.' It's the only answer I have.

'What does that even *mean*?' The bed sinks as she sits down next to me, and even though it feels like conceding, I let myself dip into Grace's shoulder.

'Do you think she's not keeping the baby because she's learnt her lesson?' It's only Grace's grip tightening around my middle that'll stop my heart from tumbling if I dare to say what's coming next out loud. 'Do you think she wishes she hadn't kept me? Is that why she's having an abortion? Cos she doesn't like being a mum?' I look at nothing but the rug and the mark I made on it the time I spilt a can of Diet Coke when we were listening to Pink and dancing our mutually appreciated hearts out.

'Izzy,' Grace says, her voice sticking on the lump in her throat as she lifts my chin with her finger so I can't look at the stain any more. 'I'm *one hundred percent* certain your mum doesn't regret having you. You're fuckin' *perfect*. Look at us,' she says, dragging me to the mirror, 'we *both* are.'

'You think?'

'I don't *think*.' Grace turns away from her reflection, holds my face in her hands. 'I goddamn *know*.'

'But maybe if Mum had said no to a baby the first time around, she'd never be in this mess.'

'Who *knows*, Izzy. She might *still* have met Daniel. Or someone *like* him. We'll never know. Thing is, she *did* have you. She *wanted* to have you. She *chose* to have you. And *god*, Izzy, the times when I'm at yours that she's told me how *proud* she is!'

'Really?'

'Really.'

And I remember, then, when I was still young enough to

go to bed earlier than Mum did, how she'd come into my room at night long after she thought I was sleeping, kneel by my bed, pull my hair from my face and whisper how sorry she was for not being a better mummy, how I was the very best thing in her life.

'Her decision is nothing to do with you,' Grace says. 'It's because of Daniel.'

There are so many reasons why Grace Izzy Ashdown is my best friend and this, right here, right now, is one of them.

FORTY-TWO

'Izzy?' Even though Mum's voice is over two hundred miles away, I can feel it on my skin, in my bones. 'Has that boy been near you? Because if he has, I swear to god I'll —'

'It's fine, Mum.' I can't talk about Jacob now. Not with her. Can't bear the thought of her knowing about those photos. About what I did in that room on that bed with that boy. 'I'm safe.'

'When Grace called me I —'

'Please,' I say.

And Mum must recognise it, the shame I feel. 'Izzy,' she says again, all caught up in tears this time, riding along the ribbons of *thank god*s that tie our words together like an old-style telephone cable. Her *thank god* that I don't hate her, her *thank god* that I'm OK.

'We *will* talk about it,' she tells me. 'When you're ready.'

I nod a kind of *maybe* that she can't see, obviously, but seems to sense.

'Just wait at Grace's,' she says, changing the subject. 'I'm coming to get you.' But there's no way I'm letting her near this town, risking her being this close to Daniel.

'It's too dangerous.' I mean because Daniel might hurt her, but there's that other side of him that scares me just as much.

210

That gentle, pleading, careful, pleasing side that knows just which words to pluck to make her knees a little weaker.

'I'm coming,' she says, like mother knows best. 'It's my job, Izzy. I'm s'posed to protect you.'

Protect? And it's funny, right, how everything can seem so much better but then one word, even one with the very best of intentions, can flip it into reverse. It's not like she doesn't mean it. Cos her voice, her voice is a gazillion years of animal instinct – that maternal drive to keep her offspring safe. But what's a gazillion years when all I wanted, all I needed, was the last six? Because if it's her job, then what? Was she on some kind of sabbatical? Where was the protection then?

I try. I swear I try not to bite, but the animal instinct's not just hers, right? And it comes, this anger, emptied of its heat so it's more bitter, like some shame-on-you disappointment, which I know is the last thing my mum, my mum who's been through Daniel's hell, needs right now. But it comes. Quietly. Though she hears it anyway.

'*Protect* me?'

'Yes.' Her voice is a Jenga tower.

'Really?' My doubt removes the bottom block.

'Really,' she says, and I can hear the topple in it. 'I'm your mum. It's what mums do.'

Six years. Of hands. Of mouths. Of hate. For Daniel. For Jacob. For me. So much of it for me.

It's not that I'm mad – there's too much lump in my throat for me to shout at her. 'And the baby? You're *protecting* that as well, are you?'

'Izzy.' Her voice is smothered by the fallen bricks, the obvious tears. 'It's not like that.'

And I could leave it. I know I could, and I should, but.

Six years.

'What *is* it like then, Mum? Like Sinitta maybe? How you got rid of her too?'

'That was different.'

'How? She needed you to look after her. Like I did. Maybe I should just be grateful a daughter's trickier to get rid of than a cat.' I pause, wondering if I should, and then I do. 'Or a baby, right? Cos it seems they're easy to get rid of too.'

'It is *not* easy,' she says.

'No? Seems to me it is. I heard you on the phone to the rescue place that time. "Lovely," you said. Like you were ordering a fucking cake. She was my cat, Mum. *My* cat, who'd belonged to *my* dad, and you got rid of her. Just like that.'

'I had to.'

'You had to? What? Because she was sick?'

'Because she was pregnant.'

'What?'

'Sinitta was pregnant.'

'All the more reason to look after her then. I mean, seriously, Mum, what kind of monst—'

'He said he'd drown them, Izzy.'

'Huh?'

'Daniel. He said he'd drown the kittens if we kept them. And then he'd drown Sinitta too.'

The silence is like Daniel with a bowl of water. Calm. Deadly.

'That's why I gave her away. I was protecting her. In my own way, Izzy, I promise I *was* protecting her.'

'And what about *me*, Mum? What about protecting *me*?'

'I'm trying,' she says. And her voice is like a red sky at night, like maybe there are storm clouds but mostly what it's made of is hope. 'I'm not going back, Izzy. Ever. You might think the shaved head thing's a gimmick, and maybe it was at the start, like it was a way of tricking myself into thinking differently. But it's made me stronger. Freed me from all sorts of crap, made me see myself differently, and not just because I'm bald.'

I might not be ready to talk but I give her an 'mmmm', so she at least knows I'm here. Listening.

'I'm sorry we stayed as long as we did. Really, really sorry. But although you know some of it, you don't know it all. He took everything. Every inch of me. But I'm getting it back, I promise you. I *am* getting it back. And he will never hurt us again.'

'OK.' It's one word. Just one word that doesn't say enough but says all that I can say because maybe it is OK. Or it will be.

'I'll come for you in the morning,' she says, this tone between us so far from normal but just far enough away from bad.

'No.'

'I'm not arguing about this, Izzy.'

'Neither am I. I'm not the only one who needs protecting, Mum.'

'There's no other option.'

But I'm thinking maybe there is.

'I know someone,' I say, ignoring how sharply she intakes her breath, which doesn't bode well, carrying on anyway because it has to be better than risking everything with her coming down here. 'There's this boy.'

Grace finally looks up at me from the book she's been pretending to read this whole time, like, *you didn't mention a boy*, and my shoulders and brows are like, *when did I have the chance?* And she's all grin then, making small circles with her finger so I'll wind up the call and spill.

'I've been sculling with him. Rowing.' This sends Grace full-on la-la because the Izzy she knows is totally couch potato. 'In the mornings,' I say to Mum, who isn't yet saying no, which I take as a bonus and plough on. 'He's really nice.'

'What's his name?' *Like that makes a difference*, I think, but whatever, cos Harry sounds super sensible and kind of posh, though Mum of all people should know anyone can be anything, no matter what they're called.

'Harry,' I say, and I know she's going to want a surname too, but we spent too much time kissing to bother with detail. So, yeah, probably not the best start to this new phase with my mum but, desperate times and all that, so I'm going to lie, only time's ticking, but maybe my brain's not. Ticking, I mean, because I keep talking and, without any proper thought, out it pops: 'His name's Harry, Mum. Harry like Styles.' And Grace practically pees herself.

'Harry like Styles?'

'Yep.'

And the three of us collapse into giggles, which feels so much closer to normal I could cry.

'So,' Mum says, when we're calmer and I can hold the phone to my ear without snorting, 'you're suggesting I let this Harry like Styles, a boy about whom I've previously heard nothing, drive all the way from Shrewsbury to Whitstable to pick you up and bring you back here?'

'That's exactly what I'm suggesting.'

Grace gives me this double thumbs up before turning away, wrapping her arms around her body so her hands are on her back, which she caresses like she's in some kind of *Love Island* sex clinch. I kick her butt, like literally kick it, and almost fall over, less because of my lack of one-legged balance and more because of the heart-busting glee I'm feeling for being in her room, by her side, kicking her butt and being so absolutely ordinary.

'I don't know if I can allow this,' Mum says. 'With everything that's happened, I just want you to be safe.'

'Trust me,' I say, and I don't know why but she does.

'OK.'

I bite down on my knuckles to stop the whoop in my chest from making a real-life noise.

'I want to meet him first though. Tell this Harry like Styles to get to the bandstand in the quarry park for seven.' Mum's voice is a *take it or leave it*.

And I'll take it, obviously, but I ask, 'Are you serious?'

'Yes, Izzy, I'm serious. If he doesn't show, or if he does and I don't trust him, I'm collecting you myself.'

'OK, OK,' I say, trying not to think of it as a test – of him, of her, of me. 'At least you'll be easy for him to spot, what with that big bald head of yours.'

Grace spits out her Coke, like, *WTF?*

I nod, like, *yeah, my mum is seriously Vin Diesel these days.*

'Seven P.M., Izzy,' Mum says, 'or *I'm* leaving at half past.'

'Harry will be there,' I say, maybe sounding like I believe it, but honestly I have no idea if he will.

FORTY-THREE

'So *that's* what you were doing all those mornings by the river.' Grace looks almost relieved. 'I was worried you'd gone totally Shropshire and taken up *fishing*!'

'What do you know about Shropshire? Or fishing? And even if I had, I reckon it's *your obsession*, not fishing, that's the issue here!' My aim is perfect – the pillow hits her square in the face! 'I mean, seriously, Grace, were you actually checking up on me at six A.M.?'

'Don't be *ridiculous*, Iz. Of course I wasn't.' Grace's mock sheepishness gives way to a smile. 'It was at *least* six thirty before I looked. Anyway,' she says, 'I was *merely* looking out for you, like I've *always* done. You know, like how I'd *call* you most mornings? Run through your *timetable* to be sure you had the right *books*? You didn't complain *then*, did you? Saved you from *thousands* of detentions, I reckon. I'm just grateful I don't have to save you from thousands of *fishing hooks* now.'

'Or lampreys.'

'You what?'

'Lampreys. One of the kids in the refuge warned me about them. Bloodsucking eels that live in the river Severn.'

'*Jesus*, Izzy.' Grace clutches her chest as the rest of her wobbles with a shiver. 'Though I guess the eels weren't the only things looking to *suck someone's face off* in Shrewsbury, were they?!'

'Ha ha.' Thing is, Grace has a point, and she knows it too.

'Oooooh, look at you, Iz – you've gone *totally* candyfloss. How sweet,' she says, winking. 'Come on then, tell all.'

And I will, I promise, but priorities, right, cos Mum insisted on this pre-pick-up meeting at seven, which only gives me an hour to explain to Harry why I ran off this morning, why I've lied about being on holiday with my mum and why I'm now in Whitstable over two hundred miles away, and would he mind, you know, despite me being a total freak and all, driving to come get me? Oh, and yes, obviously I'm still that independent girl he fell for, but Mum doesn't want me getting the train because it's too expensive, too much hassle and she just wants to know I'm not on my own and with someone who cares. And he *is* someone who cares, isn't he?

'Izzy.' And be still, my acrobatic heart, cos Harry's voice doesn't sound like a blockade when he answers the phone. 'I didn't know whether to call you,' he says, like he's the one who's done something wrong here.

'I'm sorry,' I say, and I wish that would cover it, that he could get it – everything, I mean – from those two words, and that I'd be saved from the details, from all of that nasty truth. I run my foot over the stain on Grace's rug, but like my own bruisy spots, it doesn't budge. They're part of me now. For good, I reckon. 'We need to talk,' I say.

I can hear the nerves in his 'Sure', and he must think I'm

going to end it, whatever 'it' is, and so I rush into it, the story of my life, while Harry like Styles listens quietly on the other end of the line.

And it's surprisingly easy, when I can look at the rug and not at his face – it's not too hard telling him about Daniel and the reasons why Mum and I were on the run. But the flow's dammed when it comes to explaining why I said I couldn't be with him and scarpered.

'It's kind of complicated,' I tell him. 'It's just that there've been some boys and maybe I feel like I don't —' Grace shoots me this look, like, *don't you dare. Don't you dare say you don't deserve him.* 'What I'm saying is: it's not you, Harry.'

'It's not you. It's me?' And his voice in a joke in a cliché.

'Exactly. It's not you. It's me. It's definitely me, and I'm definitely sorry, and I'll understand, you know,' I tell him, wondering if the reason he's now so silent is because he's drowning in all that heart I've just poured out down the phone, 'if you'd rather not see me any more.' I wish that maybe I *had* taken up fishing because then I'd stand a chance of reeling it all back in. 'Maybe Grace's mum can give me a lift back. I realise it's a lot to ask and I —'

'How will I know it's your mum?'

'Or maybe she'd be OK with me getting the train to London and meeting her there.'

'Will she be wearing a rose? Or holding a sign with my name on it like a taxi driver at the airport?' Harry's voice is like music when I'm focused on something else. I hear the noise of it, but the words don't register. Not fully.

'There's this woman, Kate, at the refuge – she's got a car, I think. Perhaps she could come.'

'Izzy!' Harry is louder this time. 'I'll be there for seven!'

'You'll what?'

'I'll be there for seven.'

And how I hear it is: 'I'll be there for *you*.' And it's a good job the call is only audio cos my eyes burst into a million happy tears.

'You OK?' Harry says.

And I tell him yes a thousand times because, for so many reasons, I feel like I actually might be.

'So, I'm looking for a short woman with a shaved head?' Harry clarifies when I've calmed myself enough to give him the low-down on Mum.

'And a ton of questions,' I warn him, cos Mum didn't sound like she was gonna go easy.

'I'll take my ton of answers then,' Harry says, and not for the first time, I wish he was here so I could suck his Shropshire face off!

'Thank you.' The words seem so insufficient but I say them over and over until he tells me to stop.

'This is for my benefit as much as yours, Izzy.'

'How's that?'

'Five hours in a car with you. Your mum's not the only one with questions.'

'Surely I've just told you enough of my secrets to allow me a bit of silence on the way back.'

'Nah, ah, ah. You've told me about Daniel. I want to know about *it's not you, it's me*, Izzy.'

And that poured-out heart puts a cork in it then when I think about exactly what kind of info he's after. Jacob Mansfield? But before I can tell him I've changed my mind – that Mum can come get me after all – Harry's telling me to wish him good luck, and he's gone.

FORTY-FOUR

'You heard what happened with Jacob? Harry's going to hate me if he finds out. He'll think I'm a —'

'A *what*?' Grace cuts in, and I know what she's thinking, because in those few hours she wasn't off making sweet love with Nell, we'd had this discussion over and over, after that first photo when the boys – and some of the girls! – didn't just stick it to me with Fingers but branched out into other insults too.

'He's going to think you're a *what*, Izzy?' she says again, obviously not letting it slide. 'Listen –' Grace's eyebrows lift into arches that could rival Ronald McDonald's – 'from what Max told me this morning about the *deal* Jacob made with you, it didn't sound like *you* did anything. It sounds like it was *done* to you. That's why I *had* to call your mum. There was no *consent* there. He *raped* you.'

And I totally cramp at that.

'It's a word, Izzy. The action was worse,' she says, wiping my tears before she wipes her own. 'Dumbledore?' She sees my confusion through the wet. 'He said to call something what it is, remember? Voldemort. Rape.' And maybe I wince a little cos Grace takes my hands and kisses them, a reminder of the kindness another body can bring. 'Being scared of the word makes you more scared of the thing it represents, less able to face it down. Jacob might call it all fair play or banter or some other kind of shit as disguise, but it was rape.'

And she seems so sure as she gives me her hot chocolate. There's no doubt as she holds me while I drink it. Not a slither of a *maybe I played my part in it* as she tells me over and over how sorry she is for not working out exactly what Jacob was up to.

'What he did is *not* who you are, Izzy. It *doesn't* define you. No more than what happened with Daniel *defines* your mum. I'm not saying they're not *huge shitty* things that went on, and that they won't shape you in some way, but if Harry likes you, he'll listen, and he'll get what you've been through and he'll be kind and understanding and loving and everything else you deserve.'

'That was quite a speech.' It comes out a little mean, but all Grace does is hold me tighter. 'You really think he won't mind?'

'It's not *his* to mind, is it? I'm serious. You deserve someone who's not just going to accept you for who you are and everything that's happened but someone who will *love* you all the more for it.'

'Like Nell does with you?'

'Like *you* do with me, Izzy.' Grace looks at me like, *duh!* '*Who* do you think gave me the confidence to be myself all these years?'

'What?' I don't get it.

'You've always had *so* much faith in me, this *ginormous, unshakeable* faith that I'm amazing, that I can do *whatever* I set my mind to, that I'll face down anyone who questions *who*

I am or *who* I love. You've been there for *all* of it, Izzy, and you never had *any* doubt that I'm the best.'

'That's because you are,' I tell her.

'In *your* eyes, yes. Not *everyone* has so much confidence. But that doesn't really matter, because *you* always *do*. And you're *always* telling me, never letting me forget how *awesome* I am.' She strikes her fiercest Beyoncé pose then blows me a kiss. 'I don't think I've ever even thanked you,' she says, more serious now as she sits me down on the bed. 'Not properly. So, *thank you, Izzy Grace Chambers* for being the most wonderful friend a girl could ever ask for. My life would have been *totally shit* without you.'

And in this moment, I'd one hundred percent swear Grace's sixth-sense thing is as real as her arms, which she squeezes around me with such force I can barely catch my breath. But I've never been so happy to gasp for air.

'I love you, Grace Izzy Ashdown,' I tell her when the hug eases and my body's still buzzing with the mass of love she's somehow pressed into my skin. I mean, it's probably pins and needles, but the moment's so magical I'm half expecting a unicorn to turn up and offer me a lift so I don't have to risk *that* conversation with Harry.

'I love you too,' she says, with no extra emphasis because every word is important. 'More than anything.'

I'm so tempted to ask, '*More than Nell?*', but I sit in our loosened hug instead, wondering how I can capture these last few minutes and stick them in a bottle to sit, rainbow-coloured and proud, with the Jar of Sunshine I'm going to rescue in the morning.

FORTY-FIVE

'Harry like Styles is coming to get you!' Mum called to tell me last night after her meeting with Harry, and I'm still verging on nervous gaga this morning when Grace bumps open the door into her room with her hip, bearing a tray with a two-course breakfast she presents like she's the winner of *Bake Off.* 'Ta-da!'

'Pot Noodle and toast? Really?' Even by Grace's standards, this is unconventional.

'*The breakfast of queens!*' she says, balancing the tray on my legs sprawled across the bed before budging me over so we can share. '*Actually*, it's the breakfast of a daughter whose dad forgot to order his Tesco delivery. But it'll do.'

There's no doubting it's kind of weird, but it fits, because I'm feeling kind of weird too, like these two different parts of me are about to collide and the reaction will be either dazzling or totally catastrophic.

'And how far has fair *Harry* progressed on his journey?' Grace asks, the sound of his name sparkling like a Christmas bauble as she kitten-licks Nutella from the toast.

'I'm surprised you're not tracking his every movement on Find My Friend by now!'

'I only do that with very *special* people,' she says with this joke-psycho voice and these joke-psycho eyes, which she drops before saying for the millionth time how sorry she is, you know, that she hadn't figured out Daniel for the total a-hole that he is.

'It's not your fault,' I say, nerves curbing my hunger but picking at the noodles anyway cos, like Grace keeps telling me, I need to keep my strength up.

'For all that *kissing* you're going to be doing!' she says, because that and the drive to Shropshire are all she thinks are on the agenda today.

I haven't told her about the Jar of Sunshine, that the beads are the main reason I'm here. That my reunion with her may have been the best, but it wasn't planned, whereas sneaking into Daniel's was.

And for all the same reasons – 'You can't do it, Izzy! Don't you dare, Izzy! It's too dangerous, Izzy!' – I haven't mentioned that I've had another message from him this morning, a photo of my jar in the garden next to the forget-me-nots we planted when his mother died three years ago, the same morning we first tried to leave. When he'd cried pretty much non-stop for five days, wishing, he said, that he'd seen his mother more, helped his mother more, loved his mother more.

'It's too late now,' he'd whispered, and I remember thinking how it may have been too late for his mother, but it wasn't too late for us. How maybe all this regret was what he needed to make his promises to Mum and me come true.

'I thought after Dad…He was so…She never stood a…' Daniel started but then stopped when he got home from the funeral he'd insisted on going to alone, bending himself like a little boy into Mum's lap on the sofa, the smear of his tears on her shirt and his hands clinging on to her hips. 'You're all I have now,' he said. 'You're everything I've got.' And the sobbing turned his voice into a stuck record. 'Never leave me. Never leave me. Never leave.'

We'd only met his mother the once, when she came to the wedding, looking, as she arrived, nothing like the 'mean and mousy' woman Daniel had described. When she left only an hour into the reception, I watched Daniel follow her across the road and on to the slopes leading down to the sea, saw how he grabbed at her elbow when she reached for her car door, pushed his face down into hers like he might spit in it and then, catching my stare, kissed her cheek instead. And maybe she sensed the switch in him too because she also cast a glance in my direction, but I was too far away, too much of a stranger to understand the way she looked at me. I wonder now if it was sympathy.

In this most recent picture, the Jar of Sunshine stands yellow amid the purplish blue of the flowers, with a small sign laid on the soil: *I'll never forget you, Isabel.*

If it was anyone but Daniel this might be a goodbye, an I-know-you're-not-coming-home-but-I'll-remember-what-we-had kind of farewell. But every word of Daniel's feels like it's been dipped in acid, like he corrodes the meaning of things so you can't rely on your gut to understand.

'Izzy!' Noodles slither from the tray to the duvet like tiny frantic snakes as Grace leaps from the bed to the window. 'A car's *just* pulled up outside.' The squeaking of her fingers rubbing at the cloud of her breath on the glass is sort of comedy, but I'm suddenly too breathless to laugh. 'Ooooh, Izzy Grace Chambers, isn't Harry *like Styles* a *dream*!' And she's waving at him then, giving him the best of her smiles, as she signals we're on our way down.

'Hey,' he says at the front door.

I can feel Grace's eyes on me, watching how I handle Harry's obvious pleasure in seeing me, how my body yields to his hand on my back, how I don't wait for him to make the next move but tilt my head and ask him, 'May I?' and press my lips to his when he says yes.

'That was *fast*,' Grace says, and I think she means the kissing, but she rolls her eyes, like, *duh*. 'The *drive*, Izzy. Not everything's about your blossoming *romance*, you know! Lovely to meet you, Harry *like Styles*.'

His eyes wrinkling with the confusion make him even cuter as he shakes Grace's hand.

'I've heard *a lot* about you,' she says, and I turn back towards the house, sort of wishing she'd scarper but mostly pleased it's so clear she approves.

'So how soon are you two *lovebirds* heading off?' Grace asks when she's made Harry a coffee and grilled him on last night's 'interview' with Mum.

'Soon,' Harry says with mild panic when he glances at his watch. 'I promised your mum I'd get you back as early as possible. I also promised I'd take lots of breaks during the drive. And she'd rather we weren't driving in the dark.'

'Afraid your hands might wander,' Grace says, then looks at me awkwardly, like maybe that kind of joke is all sorts of wrong.

It's OK, I smile.

Harry is all red cheeks and bumbling 'no's as I tell him to

ignore her, that she's got a one-track mind cos she hasn't seen her girlfriend in weeks.

'And *whose* fault is that, Izzy?' But her fake pout bursts into a beam since she's all set for seeing Nell this evening, especially as her mum is feeling bad about missing any clues for what was going on with me.

'Can you tell Nell I'm sorry?' I say to Grace when Harry and I are leaving.

'She's cool, Iz. She can hardly blame *you* for what happened that night, can she?'

'It's not just that night though, is it?' The inside of my bottom lip bleeds metallic guilt between my teeth as I figure out how best to put it. 'I don't think I've ever really been that kind towards her.' And Grace has this sad look that confirms it. 'I really am sorry,' I tell her. 'I felt like I was losing you though.'

'You'll *never* lose me, you idiot. You're my goddamn number-one girl.'

'Goddamn it, you're right. See you soon, yeah?'

'Soon,' she says, thrusting the bag she's leant me into my lap, shutting the car door and checking I've done up my seat belt. 'Let me know when you're ho—' She checks herself, realising, I suppose, that Mum and I are still in-betweeners, not yet belonging anywhere, not yet sure where it's safe to call home. She blows me kisses from the pavement until we reach the end of the road.

'Ignore him,' I tell Harry when his satnav tells him to turn right. 'We have to go somewhere else before we leave.'

God knows what Mum said to him because even the thought of delaying our journey seems to send him into some kind of fluster. 'I promised we'd get back as quickly as possible.'

'I understand, but this won't take long.' I place my hand over his on the gearstick. 'I'm not leaving Whitstable without my Jar of Sunshine. If you won't come with me to get it, then you may as well just drop me here.'

FORTY-SIX

It smells of him, the house. Of his aftershave and the bacon he'll have eaten for breakfast, like he does every Saturday after parkrun, where if he's not running, he's volunteering, standing on the slopes cheering on the slow starters with his high fives. Those encouraging hand slaps of his. Daniel is good like that, you see. At being one thing for them and another thing for us.

People say, don't they, that if they were veggie, the thing they'd miss most would be bacon. But here, in the fat-scented ghost of it, I'd happily eat anything but.

'You sure he's not home?' Harry's voice is a thumping heart in the quiet, as I push the front door to behind us, wiping my feet on the mat even though we're not staying, even though I'd love to screw Daniel's rules and enter the house in a blaze of mess and dirt. The muscle memory's greater than the rebellion, I guess. He has us set in his ways.

'We watched him leave,' I remind Harry for, like, the tenth time, purposefully not copycatting his whispers. And anyway, you can feel it when Daniel's here, that atmosphering thing he does, the temperature not exactly changing but the air thinning, like a castaway once described how it is at the top of a mountain, how without that oxygen, you can never feel one hundred percent safe because the truth is that your body's slowly dying. 'You saw. He left for writing group. We've got a couple of hours at least.'

When we pulled up outside, I went totally movie, slumping down in the back of Harry's car, shoving a cap of his brother's I'd found in the footwell on my head and peering through the rear window at the front of the house, waiting for Daniel to appear.

Harry pretended to play on his phone. 'That him?' he said, when Daniel opened the front door. And I could hear the surprise, the *he doesn't look like someone who…*

So, before he could say it: 'Clooney, right?'

'Totally,' Harry said, watching my stepdad in full-on charm offensive as the neighbour, Bob, wrestled with an overstuffed bin bag, Daniel making a show of putting his rucksack on the pavement so he could lift the lid of the bin before catching the yoghurt pot and envelope that had escaped through the split in the sack, clearly not reprimanding Bob for not recycling, not telling him how lazy he is, how selfish, how, *Jesus Christ, you're so stupid sometimes*, not taking the recyclables and putting them in Bob's bed as a reminder of why we have these ways of doing things. None of that. Daniel was all smiles for the neighbour and strokes for the cat.

All the while, Harry was watching him, and I knew what he was thinking: *Can this Daniel really be the same Daniel as the one who said all the words and did all the things?*

'He's a good actor,' I said. 'Not just for money, but all the way through.'

I saw the nod of Harry's head through the gap between the

headrest and the front seat, totally subtle so as not to attract Daniel's attention.

'I know,' Harry said.

And I think he does – know how good an actor Daniel is, I mean. Because although Harry's big, taking up the bulk of this boxy hallway, it's like in sneaking here into this house, he's lost the brawn of the river, like even the idea of Daniel is enough to shrink him down.

'Your mum would kill me for letting you do this.'

What I don't say is: '*You know if he finds us, Daniel will kill us first.*'

'Grab that, will you?' I say instead, pointing at the *happiness* picture on the wall, which Harry slides from its hook, his eyes all *can we go now?* But I'm up the stairs before he can try again to persuade me.

'Izzy.' His voice is a searchlight, but dimmed, like a candle maybe, as his feet creak on the treads.

He follows me to my bedroom, which is almost but not quite how I left it. Everything is straighter, neater, no dust, and my T-shirts are folded into piles, my shoes stacked in their pairs, my duvet pressed perfectly flat across my bed. I can picture him doing it, casting his eyes over the photos of Grace and me on the wall, as his hands made everything look better.

'There, there,' he'd say to Mum sometimes, as if people who aren't 1950s mothers in films actually say that to each other. And he'd stroke her hair and her back, smoothing out the creases of his anger, willing her skin to yield to his apology as much as it did to his hurt.

'Come on, Izzy.' Harry is literally pacing, his trainers leaving specks of dried mud on the carpet. Evidence. I'm on my knees then, pinching the flecks of dirt between my nails, dropping them into my palm, flushing them down the toilet, the rushing water sounding like a roar in the otherwise silent house, turning Harry's face a colour not far off porcelain, and he's wiping his hands on his jeans like he wishes he could flush away his fingerprints too.

He follows me back across the landing and into my room, hand on my shoulder, like he's ready to pull me out of here. I mean, it's obvious, but I don't point out the smallness of the place, how if Daniel were to come home, he'd only need to stand at the bottom of the stairs, and we'd be trapped.

'Don't worry,' I say, but it's as much for me as for Harry now, and he must pick up on that fault line in my tone because his energy's ramped up a notch, his eyes flitting from wall to window to door like he's sure any second it's gonna blow.

'Harry, chill!' But my heart's like hailstones against my chest as I reach up to the shelf in my wardrobe where my Jar of Sunshine should be but isn't. 'We're not doing anything wrong. This is *my* room. *My* stuff.' Even I've dropped to a whisper now.

Harry's not stupid – he gets the shift, stands guard behind the curtain like some old guy on neighbourhood watch.

'Can we get out the back?' he asks.

I look at him, like, *what? Now?*

He shakes his head. 'If I see him out the front.'

From where I'm climbing up on my desk chair

double-checking the wardrobe, even though it's obvious the jar isn't there, I nod, *sure*, but don't mention the fences we'd have to climb or the bushes we'd have to push through cos Harry seems freaked out enough already.

There are Mum's Judy Blumes and the picture of Grace and Sinitta but definitely no jar. 'It's not here.' And maybe I stamp my foot or something because suddenly I'm wobbling and Harry's catching me as I fall.

'Bloody hell, Izzy!' he says, but his voice is a this-is-the-last-thing-we-need-right-now kind of giggle, and he kisses me, proper full on with lips and tongues, the first since he arrived, and for a minute the room is painted yellow instead of that orangey red.

Because I kiss him too. Like, really kiss him. Like, kiss him with my mouth, and my hands and my whole entire body kiss him, feeling it everywhere, not just in my skin and my bones but around them too, like the kiss is everything, not just something we're doing but what we're made of and what we're standing on and what we're breathing. As if our holding and hoping can wipe away all the words Daniel said and all the things Jacob did. Because I swear I can feel it, Harry's desire – not a sexual desire, though, yeah, that's in there too, I guess, but a desire for making things good. For me. It's about me more than it's about him and that's what makes me want to keep kissing Harry more.

And more.

And more.

FORTY-SEVEN

'Shit.'

It's not clear who says it first, Harry or me, because we both hear it, the noise from downstairs that meteorites its way into that perfect kiss, catapulting us from our high to high alert, jumping us apart so we're dead still and listening for another sign.

'Do you —'

I cover Harry's mouth with my hand and give him these eyes, like, *silence!* And that bubble we'd made of hope is suddenly dripping with fear.

Every one of our breaths is a firework.

'Did you —' Harry says into my fingers, and I nod because, yeah, I heard it a second time too.

I imagine Daniel planning his next move, or maybe not planning anything, just waiting at the bottom of the stairs for when I appear. Thing is, I'm stuck, like literally cannot lift my feet to edge any closer to the door.

Harry though, Harry slides to the window, shrugs that there's nothing to see and is back by my side, with his arm against my arm and his hip against my hip and his lips against my ear, whispering, 'We need to get out of here.'

I know, right, but how and where? And we don't have the Jar of Sunshine so no. I'm not leaving without it.

I take the *happiness* picture from Harry, grasp it so tight my knuckles turn the yellow-red of rhubarb and custard sweets. When I jolt my head towards the door, Harry's eyebrows are like, *really?* But we don't have a choice, and maybe it's the inevitability of it, of some kind of showdown, or maybe it's this raging need, like when I was on the riverbank and those boys were rapping about rape like it was all just bants, yeah? Like how my blood got hotter and all I really, really wanted was to burn them down. I raise the picture, the sharp corner of the frame ready to strike, and make my way to the landing.

We stand like this, side by side, hearing only our hearts and the air we take in and blow out, take in and blow out, as we wait.

For a sign.

For a noise.

For a man.

Nothing.

And my grip becomes loose, and my heart becomes slower, and Harry and I give each other this look, like, *what idiots!* And I take a step down, and then…

Something.

It's tiny. Like, so tiny you'd never normally notice it, but that's how Daniel works, right, with these small things that seem like nothing until, all of a sudden, the shit couldn't hit the fan any harder.

Harry points at the front door only a few feet from the bottom of the staircase. We could run for it. Then there's this slither of a shadow on the sitting-room carpet and Harry looks at me, like, *move*, but I'm back in Jacob's room, unable to say yes or no, my body just waiting for whatever's going to happen to happen.

'Go,' Harry whispers, but the whisper's not silence and it turns the shadow into clatter and chaos, and Harry's not waiting now but reaching for my wrist as he stumbles down the stairs, staying upright, but only just, bringing me down with him, stretching for the latch to the door but it's too late because there are footsteps and a 'What the...?' as a rolling pin comes flying from the sitting room, catching his head and, with the impact and the shock of it, Harry stumbles and falls to the floor.

FORTY-EIGHT

'Who on earth?'

The voice is a stranger's. A woman's. Chocked full of her own shock and fear.

Harry sees her first, and the heave of his chest, the way he sinks into the door, it's not surrender but relief. We're fine. For now.

But who the hell is it?

'Isabel?' the woman says, lowering the hand mixer with which she was ready to go into battle.

That face, though I can't place it, isn't so much of a stranger as I'd thought.

'I'm sorry –' the free hand she reaches down to Harry is heavily lined and ringless – 'for the rolling pin.' And though her voice is as old as the rest of her, it's also the uneasy shyness of a child hiding behind her mother's legs.

''S cool,' Harry says, refusing her offer of a helping hand up. 'I'm good, thanks. God knows what you might be planning to do with the beater attachment on that mixer!'

'I'm sorry,' she says again, not registering his smile, his joke. The repetition has the same familiarity as her face. Only, her face reminds me of Daniel and her sorries remind me of Mum.

''S OK, honest.' Harry's up on his feet, and the woman, who must be in her seventies, shrinks a little as he moves towards her. 'I was just gonna take that for you,' he says, minding his step, filling his voice with no hard feelings, and she hands her weapon over.

'You *are* Isabel, aren't you?'

'Izzy, actually.' It's kind of harsh, the way I correct her, but these things count, right?

'Of course. Izzy.' And there's an understanding in how she says it. And in how she lowers her eyes, kind of awkward, kind of sad – there's a sort of apology in there too. 'You've grown since…'

'Since?'

'Daniel and Stephan—' She stops herself. 'Daniel and *Steph's* wedding. But I wasn't there for long.'

And there she is, in this memory played out like one of those Boomerang videos on Instagram, dipping away, turning her cheek from Daniel as he switched from rage to tender when he saw that I was watching.

'You're Daniel's mum?'

She nods, like that same uneasy child admitting something she thinks could get her into trouble.

'But he said you were —' And it's me who stops myself now.

'We hadn't seen each other in a long time,' she says without leaving a gap between my speech and hers, and I can't tell if she's making conversation or saving me from telling the truth.

Harry looks at me, like, *there's no time for family reunions, yeah?*

But I shake my head as soft as I can – so soft that she might miss it. But, like Mum, she seems fine-tuned to every gesture and agrees that, really, it's probably best that we go.

'Daniel says there have been some…' she tiptoes across the word, 'issues.'

Harry's eyes roll in a now-that's-what-I-call-an-understate-ment kind of disbelief. 'Is that what he calls them?'

And I give him this look, like, *don't*.

But he shakes his head. 'You know what he's done? To Izzy and her mum?'

'I can imagine.' Her voice is a flash flood filling the room with regret.

'But you're staying here anyway.' And I know he doesn't mean it, but Harry's words are a gentle attack.

'He's my son.'

'He's my husband,' Mum had said in the hours after that first time, when I'd held a warm flannel against her arm.

It's kind of amazing, and kind of scary, the ties, the binds of love.

'My jar.'

'Follow me,' Daniel's mum says, wincing slightly every time her left foot presses against the floor.

'Are you OK?'

'Yes,' she says. And *I've* said the same when I've obviously been the furthest from OK you can be.

'Shall I leave you my number?' I ask her, going to find some paper and a pen in the drawer.

'Best not.' And her voice is an acceptance of her position. 'You know what he'd do if he found it.'

When she comes back from the far end of the garden,

where we planted the forget-me-nots after she didn't actually die, the jar is warm in her hands. And although I know it's just where it's been lying in the sun, what I know too is that the heat is its power. That I was my dad's sunshine and that even if he's somewhere else, somewhere maybe 149.6 million kilometres away, he still feels me, like I still feel him. That love can carry that distance even if it has to be kept in a jar.

'Come on,' I say.

Harry's eyes are like, *are you sure we should leave her?*

My shrug won't say it, but what I mean is: *we can't make her come.*

'Quickly,' I tell Harry, taking the page Daniel cut from my book from its frame and putting it in the bag, pulling my shoes on to my feet and leaving my key right there. Because I don't want it. I don't need it. This house is not my home and I'm not coming back to it. Ever.

I hug her then, this woman whose son changed everything.

'Good luck,' Daniel's mum says, leaning in, holding tight. 'Be well.'

FORTY-NINE

'Sweets!' Harry says, shoving a packet of Starbursts in my face as we trundle around Tesco Express looking for the perfect post-shock sugar top-up. 'My nan lobbed six sugar cubes in her tea when she heard my cousin Eve had been caught nicking a kilo of chicken wings from KFC. Medicinal, she said!'

So I grab three Freddos cos, seriously, who hasn't been waiting their entire life for a medical reason to gorge on chocolate frogs?

'Three? Really? You think that's wise?' Says a voice at my side.

And I hadn't been wrong then, when I thought I spotted Jacob as we got out the car. Now here he is in the sweet aisle, looking anything but.

'I've seen that belly. Felt it too. Eh, Izzy?'

And there it is again, the voice of broken happy-ever-afters because, honestly, I was really starting to believe maybe Harry and I were heading for some kind of sunset, but then in comes Jacob and all I'm heading for is shame.

'Who's this then? He's why you came over all frigid in the park yesterday, is he?'

And though he's not biting, Harry's not exactly blank about Jacob either, his eyes to the floor and his hands preoccupied with the pack of chocolate-covered Hobnobs he'd tossed into the basket just as Jacob was making himself heard.

'Lost your tongue, have you?' Jacob says. 'Maybe it's for the best, eh! Your *boyfriend* might not wanna go near it once he knows where it's been.'

And my chest is a broken lift shaft with my heart plummeting down, down, down.

'Her *boyfriend* might be more upset about the way you're talking to her,' Harry says, head up now – his and mine – and those rower shoulders broader as he's eyeballing Jacob, who's all shrugs and *just saying*s. 'Dick,' Harry mutters as Jacob, clearly not giving a shit, struts away.

'Mega dick,' I concur, but the thing is, though we're smiling, that near-escape adrenaline rush we were buzzing on has nosedived and the heat of that sunset we were destined for has turned from a reddish kind of fire to a palish kind of meek.

'It's fine,' I snap at the man who comes over to help when the stupid self-scanning machine doesn't recognise the Freddos. 'I don't want them anyway. Shit!'

The old woman behind me in the queue tuts when I'm further delayed cos I realise I've lost Mum's purse.

'Here,' Harry says, leaning across and pressing his card to the contactless reader while the realisation that the purse may have fallen out my bag at Daniel's sinks from my head down through the rest of my body.

'That a friend of yours?' And I can hear it, how Harry didn't want to ask but really couldn't stop the words as we leave the shop, and while he's normally so easy-going, now he's all hurried steps, one hand holding the bag and the other shoved hard into his pocket. Difference being, he'd reached for mine on the way in.

'Not reall—' But I come to a standstill. Harry doesn't even notice because he's a few feet ahead, already at the car.

Daniel.

Leaning against a lamp post like some romcom hero waiting for his girl. But when I double-take, he's gone, no trace of him, no back of his head, no flash of the white shirt he was wearing this morning. Nothing. So maybe it's the panic from seeing Jacob that makes it seem as if Daniel's still looming, still atmosphering in my head.

I wonder if it will always be like this. If Daniel's face will forever appear in a crowd, like the opposite of one of those magic drawings you get on the internet – stare hard enough and you see something you totally missed at first glance.

And there's a nudge of understanding then. Why Mum doesn't want his baby. Because most likely she'll see Daniel's face in strangers like I do and couldn't cope with seeing it in her own child's too. Not to mention that cord that would tie them, like mother to baby, but mother to ex, him using it to tug at her, pull at her, and they'd always be bound.

'Can we just go?' I say to Harry, as I climb into the car. Not mentioning Daniel. Not mentioning Jacob, just reaching for my Jar of Sunshine, rolling one of the beads between my fingers, feeling its heat.

FIFTY

When he's not changing gear, Harry keeps a hand on my knee. Even when, half an hour into the drive, I tell him everything. The party. The photo. The blackmail. He keeps his hand on my knee, and I keep my eyes on the road. Because no way I can look at Harry's face as he hears all that dirty history I have with Jacob, all that proof of me being nothing like that girl he met on the river. More silent. More still. More caught in the current instead of forging a dam.

'You're not saying anything,' I say, and my head actually feels like what brains look like in photos, a mash or maze of minced beef totally incapable of thought.

'I'm not *not* saying anything,' Harry says. 'I'm just letting you talk.'

And that's it then – we fall into this gap, where he's not *not* saying anything and I'm not *not* saying anything, but neither of us says anything more.

Until.

'You know what Jacob is, don't you, Izzy?'

'A dick?'

'Not just any dick though, right?'

'A mega dick,' we say in unison.

And for the first time since I told him, I catch Harry's eye.

Time passes. We drive on, away from Jacob and Daniel and maybe even from shame.

'Pass me a biscuit,' he says. 'I need a Hobnob.'

And my eyebrows must be like, *a Hobnob, eh?* cos Harry's laughing then, and I wonder if it's real, this dismissal of my past like it genuinely counts for shit.

'Oops, sorry, this one's broken.' The crumbs spill over my lap as I try to keep the damaged biscuit in the packet and wiggle out another in a perfect piece.

'Just pass it over.' Harry reaches his hand across the gearstick. 'I don't care if it's broken. I'll take a Hobnob any way it comes. I love Hobnobs. They're my thing, you know. Like if I'm stressed, all I wanna do is eat Hobnobs.'

'You saying you're stressed?' And my heart stands still as the car moves onwards. I'd thought this was going quite well.

'Not being funny but you did just make me break into some psycho's house and steal a Jar of Sunshine!'

'Yeah, sorry 'bout that.'

'It's all right now. I have *you*, right?'

'Yes,' I say, trying so goddamn hard not to beam.

'*And* I have Hobnobs. God, I love them. Like, really, really love them.'

'I can tell.'

'Come on then, Izzy. Tell me something you really, really love.'

And in my head I'm like, '*I know it's crazy, Harry, but I might just really, really love...*' Don't even think it, Izzy. Don't even think it.

'*Desert Island Discs*,' I say.

'Ah, of course,' he says. 'You think your thing for *Desert Island Discs* is as big as my thing for Hobnobs?'

'Whatever, Harry. Let's not get into how big your thing is or isn't, yeah?'

'Izzy!' A spray of biscuit on the dashboard.

'Seriously, you need to take more control of your Hobnob!'

'Leave my Hobnob out of this, young lady.'

'You're the one who started it. But yes, I do think my thing's as big as your thing. Maybe even bigger. Funnily enough, what with your penchant for broken Hobnobs, if I had to choose eight tracks to sum up my life, one of them would be "Broken Biscuit".'

'Huh?'

'It's a song, Harry! By Sia?'

But he obviously has no clue so I cue it up on Spotify, turn up the volume on my phone and let Sia's words run into the cracks where I too am broken, willing myself to look at my boyfriend – he did call himself that, didn't he! – to see if he gets it, how gentle he needs to be with this smashed-up soul of mine.

'It's nice,' he says, when the song's done and he's given it a moment's silence out of respect for it being one of my favour-ites. 'But I'm not sure you should have it on the island.'

And seriously, it's scary how quickly respect can crumble.

'Erm, you know this is *my* selection, Harry. This isn't *our* mega dicks list – this is one of *my* actual *Desert Island Discs*.'

'Yeah, yeah, I totally get that, Iz, but these are the songs you might have to live with forever.'

And I nod, like, *duh*, cos I'm the *Desert Island Discs* expert here, remember.

'You might feel like a broken biscuit at the moment but isn't it a bit, I dunno, pessimistic to have it as part of your lifelong theme tune?'

I sit there for a bit, looking at the cat's eyes disappearing beneath the car. 'FYI, I'm not *not* saying anything. I'm just thinking.' I think. 'And anyway, it doesn't have to be forever – you know, some castaways are invited back for a second go. Maybe in twenty years *I* won't be broken any more and I'll change "Broken Biscuit" for something else.'

'Twenty years? Really? You're going to take twenty years to not feel like a broken biscuit?'

What can I say to that? Who knows how long it takes to recover from these things?

'It actually *might* take you twenty years if you're listening to this every day. I'm serious,' Harry says, when I concede with a quiet kind of laugh. 'Sia might have this amazing voice, but you have to admit that she makes being broken sound a bit, well, a bit of a lost cause.'

'And it isn't?'

'No!' Harry checks the rear-view mirror then chucks a smile at me as we pull into the service station. 'You know what my dad gave me for my eighteenth birthday?'

'A bottle of whisky? A newspaper from the day you were born?'

'No. A broken bit of pottery.'

'Jesus, gold star to your dad for that one!'

Harry parks up, puts on the handbrake and unplugs his

seat belt so he can turn to face me full on. 'It had been broken, but someone put it back together with gold.'

'Gold? On a smashed-up bit of china?'

'It's a Japanese art apparently. *Kintsugi*. And I'm probably saying it wrong, but it's the philosophy that's important.'

'The *philosophy*?' And my smile is a tease but, honestly, Harry just gets more attractive by the minute.

'Yes, Izzy, the philosophy. Because the reason they do it, piece it together with gold, is because they believe that nothing is ever truly broken.'

'But doesn't it make the cracks look more obvious?'

'Nah. It makes them look more beautiful,' he says, and even though the gearstick and the handbrake and the Hobnobs are in his way, Harry goes right ahead and kisses me right here in the services car park, where I let the broken parts of me begin to glimmer with gold.

FIFTY-ONE

I'm sorry, Sia, but you're out of here. Sure, I'm an independent woman and all that and *my* discs are *my* discs, but a girl's gotta be up for some compromise, and if that compromise comes with one of those heart-searing kisses then who am I to say no?

Because Harry was on to something with that song, like when I'm on my island, when I'm all alone and literally fighting for my life, do I really want something that reinforces Daniel and Jacob's power, or do I want something that's going to make me whoop? So fight-talking Katy Perry's in. Seriously, her track has me nailed.

Almost.

Actually, it has the hope for me nailed. Like, I'm not quite there yet, but make this my anthem and I might well be. From sitting to standing. From quiet to thunder. From biting my tongue to magnificent, fire-dancing 'Roar'.

Just listening to it gets me morphing. It's totally different from listening to Sia, when that's all we did – listen, I mean. Cos it's like Harry said: 'Broken Biscuit' is nice, kind of beautiful, but it's also kind of sedentary. When we play 'Roar', it's a whole other story. The music, the words, they do exactly what desert island music needs to do: they time-travel you. And yeah, I'd always thought they should time-travel you back to a place you've already been, to a memory you've already made, but this is the opposite. It propels me forward.

When it starts, what is it, piano? Whatever, it immediately sounds kind of happy because the past is already the past and Katy Perry's already become what she wanted to be: a fighter, a champion, a butterfly, a bee. And, yeah, it might all be cliché, but cliché is cliché because it's true, right? Because it works. Like the muscle memory that made me stick to Daniel's rules, this is the lyric memory that might just help me break them.

Harry sings too. Like, top-of-his-voice sings. And, like me, he's awful, but sod it, cos we might be awful but we're also great. Road-tripping monumental kind of great, roaring our hearts out as the song attaches itself to these few hours in the car, already making it a place for me to draw power from when I need to remind myself of my fire.

'Do you think we'll be back in time to go out on the river?'

'Today?' Harry says.

And I know what he's thinking – my mum will be waiting – but this charge I have from singing, it's too much of a force to just go sit in a refuge for the rest of the day.

'Half an hour, that's all. I'll message Mum now. She won't mind.'

'I dunno, Iz,' Harry says. 'She seemed super keen to have you there as soon as possible.'

'Being half an hour late isn't gonna kill anyone, is it?'

'S'pose.' His eyes flit to the time on the display. 'I'd just rather get you back, Izzy. Your mum…' he doesn't seem to know what to say, 'she wasn't messing around when she laid down the rules. And rule number one was straight home.'

'Well, we already broke that.'

'Yeah, and that didn't exactly turn out perfectly, did it?'

'I got the jar, didn't I? We're alive!'

'Ha! Because it's always a good sign when you're pleased to come out of something alive.' He's laughing, but Harry's voice is the huge exhale of a near miss. 'She's pretty fierce, your mum. Like you.' And he gives me this smile, like, *believe it*. 'Knows what she wants.'

'And what she doesn't want.' He hears it then, the betrayal of my thoughts. And it's not like I wanted to say it. It's not even like I wanted to think it. I was happy thinking about being a lion and taking over the world. But it lurks somewhere just beneath every other thought I'm having, this constant reminder of Mum's choice. And, honestly, I understand the reasons why she doesn't want this baby. His baby. They make complete sense, and if it was anyone else, I swear I wouldn't judge. But maybe because it's my mum, I am. Judging, I mean. Because I know she could pull it off. She could be the kind of mum she was to me before Daniel came along. She could make it work.

'Izzy?'

'It's nothing.' But the tears I've missed with the wipe of my wrist prove otherwise.

'Whassup?'

'It's my mum.'

Harry's like, *uh-huh*, as if this conversation is like any other normal conversation.

'She's pregnant.' And before Harry can even think of congratulations, I say, 'She's having a termination', rushing through the word like I used to rush through chocolate biscuits when Daniel wasn't home in some weird belief that if he wasn't there to witness it, they wouldn't count. Their moment on my lips would not be forever on my hips. But this isn't a biscuit. It *is* forever though. Either way, this decision is definitely for forever.

'And you don't think she should?' Harry makes a whole load of effort to sound neutral.

'It's the woman's right to choose.' The opinion was far more convincing when it came from Grace.

'I'm sure it hasn't been an easy decision.'

I get what he's doing, but I say, 'And you'd know, would you?'

'Yeah,' he says, still in that voice like he's used to this, like this isn't something that happens to other people, like this is something he's talked about before. 'I do.'

I don't say anything.

'You know, you're not the only one with history, Izzy.'

And this time it's Harry who keeps his eyes forward, as he reveals that his closet has skeletons of its own.

FIFTY-TWO

'She wasn't really my girlfriend.' And it's not that he sounds ashamed, but there *is* something that's different in Harry's voice now, a fragility maybe, something that doesn't quite fit with those muscles in his rower's arms that look like nothing could possibly hurt him. 'We'd been out a few times, with other mates and that, just for drinks and to a club and, you know...'

And I know, but I'm not sure I want to. The image of Harry and the girl before, the girl who wasn't really his girl-friend but who, you know...

'We weren't exactly careful.' And those breaths he takes, how he swallows, and that shake of his head, like he's been over it so many times, but nothing ever changes that one moment of being not exactly careful. I just want to reach over and hold him. 'I told her I wouldn't come inside her,' he says, daring to look at me then, like, *too much information?* Which maybe it is, but I want to hear it anyway.

'It's OK,' I tell him, and his shoulder drops under the touch of my palm.

'She couldn't stop crying after, and I was convinced she was overreacting, because what are the chances? I mean, my aunt and uncle were trying for ages, IVF and everything, and I told Kiera that, but she was so mad at me by then because, like I

said, I'd promised. And she swore if she was, you know…
Well, it'd all be my fault, wouldn't it?'

'And she was? Pregnant, I mean?'

'Yeah,' he says, like he still can't quite believe it.

And neither can my heart, which sits in my throat like a
boiled sweet, kind of small and hard and sticky.

'Crazy, innit? How easy it can happen. Can you pass me
another Hobnob?' And what's crazy is how Harry's talking
about a baby and then he's talking about a biscuit. 'Sorry,' he
says, clocking my disbelief. 'I told you, I eat when I'm stressed,
that's all.' So I pass him two and he goes on. 'I know how it
sounds. Like I was a dick.'

'Mega dick,' we say with perfect timing, and my boiled-
sweet heart slips back into my chest and begins to beat again.

'Complete and utter,' he says. 'So, a few weeks later, I get a
text saying she needs to see me. We met in the park, and she
was already crying before she pulled out the test and, god,
those two lines. They looked so harmless. That was it then,
wasn't it? The rest of our lives.'

'What did you say?'

'Shit.' And he looks at me, like, *honest*. 'I said "shit". A lot.
There were some sorries in there too, but I think for the next
week or so pretty much the only word that came out of my
mouth was "shit".'

'And what about…?' I remember her name's Kiera, but it
feels weird to say it, like an intrusion almost. 'What about
your not-really girlfriend? What did she say?'

'All sorts,' Harry says now, pausing to listen to the satnav
telling him to take the second exit at the roundabout. 'Mostly

she was scared, I reckon. Of telling her mum and dad. At first, she said there was no way she could have an abortion.' Even though he doesn't stammer over the word, Harry's voice does drop a little as he says it. 'But over the next few days, after she spoke with her parents, she started to think differently.'

'And what did *you* want?'

'Honestly? I don't know what I wanted. I mean, if you'd have asked me a few weeks before if I wanted a baby, then obviously I'd have been, like, no way. But when it happens, you can't help wondering what it'd be like.'

'So, what did you do?'

'I worked up the balls to tell *my* mum and dad and then we all had this meeting. Can you imagine? Sitting round a table looking at the faces of the parents of a girl you had sex with after too many Jack Daniels, discussing the pros and cons of having a child. That meeting? Worst. Moment. Of. My. Life. Hands down.'

'Did anyone take the minutes?'

'The minutes?' Harry looks at me, like, *you serious?*

'The meeting! Someone always takes minutes at a meeting. Sorry, I make inappropriate jokes when I'm nervous, that's all.'

'Touché. No one took the minutes, Izzy.' But he smiles. 'It was weird, everyone talking about what would happen to "the baby". Who would look after "the baby". What "the baby" would mean for Kiera's future. Whether I could support "the baby". Where "the baby" would live. How old we'd be when "the baby" was sixteen. And then suddenly

Kiera just said she didn't want it. She wasn't ready. She didn't love me. She barely even knew me. And, yeah, she thought she'd make a good mum one day, but she didn't want to do it. Not yet.'

'What did everyone say?'

'Her mum was crying, my dad too, but Kiera's aunt had an abortion while she was at uni apparently. She has three kids now…Kiera's mum said it was Kiera's body. Kiera's life. Kiera's choice.'

'And you?'

'I think she was right. Kiera asked me straight up what I wanted, and truth is, for all my talk about stepping up and being *a man*…' Harry shakes his head, like, *whatever that means*, 'I wasn't ready to be a dad.'

'But don't you think you would have got yourself ready? That once "the baby" arrived, something would have kicked in and you'd have loved it?'

'Probably,' he says, checking his mirrors, indicating left, 'but maybe things are better this way. A baby should be wanted, don't you think?'

'I s'pose.'

'Look,' Harry says, coming to an almost standstill as we pull into town, 'it's never gonna be a decision I'm happy about, but that doesn't mean it was the wrong decision. Just means we made a mistake and we chose the path we most wanted to live with.'

Even I don't know if I'm not *not* saying anything when I sit there not saying anything at all.

'And it sounds odd but there are positives to come out of

it, Iz. I might not have had to grow up enough to be a dad, but I did grow up. My *own* dad saw to that.'

'What do you mean?' In my head, I see the kind of 'lesson' Daniel would dish out in the same situation. Maybe he feels my panic cos Harry's all 'no no no's and a hand from the steering wheel to my knee to reassure me it was nothing like that, nothing like Daniel – it was OK.

'He said I had to have more respect for women. For myself too. That talking girls into unsafe sex was…' He pauses, looks at me, like, *you can draw your own conclusion.* 'Let's just say he wasn't happy.'

'And what happened with Kiera? When she went for the…'

'Abortion?' Normal volume this time. 'We went to the appointment together. Her mum waited in the car. I'm glad I was with her. She was a bit nervous, I s'pose. But the staff were nice, and she was given these pills. She messaged me after a couple of days to say it was all over. And that was it.'

'And that was it?!' For the first time in this conversation, I feel the rise of something. 'Just like that?'

'I didn't mean it like that,' Harry says. 'Not like, *Kiera had an abortion, there we go, all done and dusted.*' And he's rising too, his hand snapping away from my leg and his voice like, *don't you judge me.* 'What I meant was, it was straightforward, not the decision exactly, but the actual procedure. And that *was* it. That was it for the idea of "the baby". That was it for Kiera and me. And, if I'm really, really honest, that was it for the sheer panic that owned me for the previous few weeks.'

At least Harry doesn't recoil when I reach for him.

'And like I said, that was also it for me being a mega dick.

For most of the time anyway,' he says, giving me this smile, like, *cut me a break, I'm really trying here.*

'Do you not think it's different for my mum though?'

'I think it's probably different for everyone, Iz. But if she doesn't want "the baby" – and from what you've told me there are good reasons why she wouldn't – then maybe it *is* the right choice for her.'

We sit with the lights on red.

'It's like Kiera's mum said. It's her body. Her life. Her choice.'

And I can feel it, the weight of Harry's expectation that I'll suddenly be one hundred percent OK with this.

The car behind us sounds its horn, and we move on.

FIFTY-THREE

We scull for exactly thirty minutes. Harry times us to be sure.

'You positive I can't drive you to the refuge?' he says when we're back at the clubhouse.

'Absolutely.' I grab Grace's bag from his locker. 'It's against the rules anyway. No one can know where it is. Safety, innit?'

He doesn't look convinced. 'It's your safety I'm thinking about.'

'What? You worried those bloodsucking eels are gonna get me, Harry?! Listen,' I say, 'I'll call my mum, tell her I'm on my way, OK?'

'OK.' He kisses me once, twice. 'Three times for luck,' he says. 'Tomorrow then.' And one more kiss goodbye.

'Tomorrow.'

And although, as he walks away, I'm already wishing tomorrow was today, I'm also glad for this time by the water, for the mum who answers the phone when I call to let her know I'm heading back from the river. Glad too for her saying 'It's fine, Izzy. Honestly, it's fine', when I repeat my sorries, meaning it this time when I tell her I respect her choice.

'I do understand, Mum, why you can't keep the baby. It's sad, but I get it. I understand.'

'I know I said it before, Izzy, but it hasn't been an easy

decision,' she says, and I think of Harry, how he wasn't being a diplomat – he was merely being fair. 'I love you so much.'

And Mum's voice is a bird's nest: all these things she's pulled from the world around us might look like a mess, but she's building with them, bringing me into the shape she's made with them, promising she'll keep me safe.

'I love you too,' I tell her, poking a stick in the river, watching how the water moves around it; how, whatever happens, the water flows on.

FIFTY-FOUR

'Isabel?'

I cling on to Grace's bag like it's one of those lifesaver rings you toss into the water if someone is drowning.

'I thought it was you.'

And even though my heart is a pneumatic drill, Daniel's voice is a tannoy linked to the sky.

'You left this behind,' he says, and even though it's quiet, his voice drowns out everything. The birds. The river. The wind.

I see his feet first, the Adidas Gazelles he's had for months but are still looking box fresh. Like the rest of him. Still so handsome. Still so George. Still so butter wouldn't melt.

'Your mum's purse, isn't it?' He's holding it out to me, the same smile he had when I first met him all those years ago when I smiled back and let him in. 'I thought you might need it.'

And his eyes too are the same, that way he can look at you, make you feel like there's no one else in the world. And it used to be a good thing. But here by the water, it feels like the scariest thing of all.

'I wouldn't have minded bringing you back, Isabel. If you'd told me you were coming. You didn't need to make that boy drive all the way up here from Kent. You should have asked.'

He drops Mum's purse into my lap when I don't take it, sits down next to me on the riverbank, watching me the whole time, still with that smile and those eyes and that confidence in his body that's so different from Harry's confidence in his.

'I got home just after you left.' He tucks my hair behind my ear like Mum used to when I was little, his finger lingering on my neck. 'Found that.' He nods at the purse on my thighs. 'My mother said you'd been.' *Your 'dead' mother*, I think. 'And what luck –' he pulls gently on my chin so my face is turned towards his – 'to see you outside Tesco like that. To be able to follow you here.' And the word 'here' sounds like a prize, like the peopleless place that it is.

'I've missed you, Isabel.' His breath is coffee and mints, those strong ones he keeps in his car. 'Did you like the pictures I sent?' And when I don't say anything, he points at Grace's bag. 'Is it in there? Your jar.'

I don't nod. I don't do anything other than just about breathe.

'I can give you a lift now, if you like.' His head cocks to the side as he waits for an answer that won't come. 'Well?' His face is frozen, his voice has dropped a few degrees, ice crystals dancing on every one of his syllables when he tells me how much effort he's made to find me, to keep me safe. 'I kept my eye on you all the way up in that boy's car. At the services too.' His thumb and forefinger make a small clamp on my jaw. 'Things got quite intense between the two of you for a while there, didn't they, Isabel?' Daniel's grip tightens, and he pulls my mouth closer to his mouth. 'All that kissing. Not for the first time from what I hear. From what I've seen.' And he pulls his phone from his pocket with his free hand. 'Harder for little sluts to keep their secrets these days, don't you think?' And there on his screen is the Fingers photo.

His laugh is so soft it tickles my nose.

It's funny what you notice when you're this near, like how Daniel's eyebrows need waxing, like how his hair isn't George's exact shade of grey.

'I'll sort that boy out for you.' He's so close, everything that comes from between his lips snakes its way between mine, filling my throat and my chest with the heavy threat of everything he's not saying, of everything he could possibly do. 'That's what good dads do, Isabel. Look after their children. Keep them from harm.'

Everything I want to say gets caught up in my throat like swallowed vomit.

'I've tried to be a good father to you, Isabel. Your mother knows that. That's why I don't understand.'

'Understand? Understand what?' I don't mean to spit them, but the hate I have is too thick with bile to keep the words down.

'Why Stephanie wouldn't want my baby.' His eyes are fixed on me.

And right here, right now is when I need Daniel not to take any of the control I've clawed back over my body, because this is when I need it to be still, to be neutral, to do the opposite of what Grace says it should, to be as silent as the rest of me and give nothing – nothing! – away.

'Your mum's pregnant.' He's barely audible. 'Isn't she?' And Daniel's voice is like that man on the news programme he listens to on the radio in the mornings, the one whose tone is calm but with an impatient edge to it when he has to repeat his question. 'Isn't she?'

'No.' I pull my head from his hold, reaching over to Grace's bag, putting Mum's purse in, taking my phone out, trying not to look too scared, not to look at any part of Daniel, not to let my stumbling thumb prevent me from unlocking it so I can dial 999.

'Liar.' He slips the unlocked mobile too easily from my palm. 'I heard you, Isabel. On the phone just now. "*I do understand, Mum, why you can't keep the baby.*"' The same impression as Jacob. And the same assumption as the rapper boys: that he has this god-given power to whittle me down. 'Tell me the truth, Isabel,' Daniel says. And then slower. Each word a bullet from a gun. 'You. Will. Do. As. I. Say.'

I feel it then, that simmering in the pit of my belly as I look him square in the eye and say, 'No.'

'No?' And his voice is a black hole, sucking in everything around him so that nothing can escape the pull of his gravity.

Except me. Because Daniel may have thought I was broken, but here I am, filled with a blast of sunshine making a *kintsugi* kind of light.

'No,' I say to all that hurt he hurled at my mother. 'No' to all those times he stole our hope. 'No' to the silence in which he buried us. 'No,' I say to Daniel. To Jacob. To those boys on the river. 'No. No. No.'

'You've found your voice,' Daniel says. 'How sweet.'

'No,' I say to his hands on my shoulders.

'No,' I say to his knee on my thigh.

'No,' I say to his mouth on my ear telling me that if my mother's going to get rid of his baby, he might just get rid of hers.

'No,' I say one last time, knowing, as always, that whatever I say is useless, because Daniel climbs on top of me and the sheer mass of him eclipses the sun.

Daniel holds me down with one hand and scrolls through my unlocked phone with the other, hitting *dial* when he sees Mum's number, muttering something about babies and bitches and 'I should have known…I should have known.'

'After everything I've done for you.' His saliva smears dirty rainbows on the screen, which he presses hard against my nose, so I hear Mum's distant 'Izzy! Izzy!' and the sudden lurch of her tears.

'Eye for an eye,' he says.

Mum's scream is a lightning bolt firing from the refuge to the river, where Daniel tosses my phone in the water and kneels over me, slowing the world on its axis and raising his hand like he's revving up for a strike.

And that thing, what they say about your life flashing before your eyes – well, it's sort of but not quite true. Nothing flashes. Everything muffles. And I begin to blank. That muscle memory luring me into flat lines and whatever will be will be. Daniel's fist comes slowly, slowly towards me, the inevitability of its punch so blunt it's like my blood vessels aren't even waiting for the blow before they cave and leak beneath my skin. The same old, same old story so familiar we both know where it ends.

My songs play somewhere beneath the water, like a farewell, distant and drowned. But then as Daniel's knuckles loom closer, I swear I see their notes pushing their way up on to the riverbank, breathing life into the beat of them, and then they rise.

And as they rise, *I* rise, my muscles pushing aside the memory of least resistance and dancing to the moon, the lagoon, the sunshine, the perfect and the roar, which have brought me here and given me a choice.

My body.

My life.

My choice.

And given a choice to trust my body's power, I say yes to it. Because Daniel may have thought Mum and I were as breakable as my necklaces, but there is light in our broken pieces and it is strong.

Daniel's pinned me with his left hand and his right hand is coming down fast; I twist my head from its path and watch it lift again, higher this time, his fingers almost catching the sun.

Yes.

I half expect to feel the heat of the Jar of Sunshine as I grab hold of it from Grace's bag. But there's no magic. When I pull it clear of the rucksack, it doesn't blind Daniel with its love light, it doesn't make him disappear, but when I pull it down harder and faster than I thought humanly possible, smacking it with all my burning power on his head, it's just enough to stun him, for him to lose his grip and drop to the side of me on to the cracks of the sun-baked mud.

I wiggle upwards, just about standing, and run.

And I run. And I run. And I run.

Along the river. Beneath the trees. Looking for someone. For anyone. I run.

My breath horror-movie heavy. My arms pumping action-movie hard. I run.

Eyes forward. Heart huge. I run.

Where are the dog walkers? The ramblers? Even the river rappers?

I run.

Away from his 'Isabel! Isabel!' Away from his 'Stop, Isabel, please!', getting louder as he runs harder and faster than me. I run.

I run where the bank expands into a field of green, but if I run into the open, there'll be nowhere to hide and so I run into the dark corridors of the weeping willows, hoping their branches will conceal me as I run not just away from but to. To the bend in the path, to the slope of the hill, to the bushes and behind, where I bury myself down in the burning sting of the nettles and hush those horror-movie heaves into slow silent breaths as I lie still and watch him appear around the corner and run.

And stop.

Daniel stops, turns full circle and smiles.

'Is-a-bel,' he sings, voice like a child in a game of hide-and-seek. 'Is-a-bel.' Turning and circling as he's seeking me out. 'Is-a-bel.' Warm. Warmer. Warmer. Hot. Hotter. Hotter. Until he's just a few metres from where the nettles lick at my ankles.

I bite on my thumb knuckle to stop the scream.

Then something flickers in the distance.

'You.'

It's not me he's talking to but someone at the top of the hill who is running down, running hard, running strong.

Mum.

I see her when she spots him, how she stands still but doesn't droop. Her feet wide. Her fists clenched. Her bald, bold head held extraordinarily high.

'*Where is she?*' Mum's voice is a rise in the sea level. '*Where's Izzy?*' she says again when he doesn't answer.

I push myself up from the ground and show her I'm here.

I run, and Mum runs, and her arms are a tent in the storm.

'Stephanie.' He smiles, and she may as well be a guest at a party cos Daniel's voice is all *how nice to see you*, and his hands are open like he's beckoning a hug. 'What happened to your hair?'

He takes a small step closer, and we take a small step back, but our steps are three-legged-race awkward and uphill and backwards so we literally can't see or feel our way out.

'Isabel told me the news. It can be our new start.' Daniel's voice is blossom as he looks at Mum's belly.

I whisper, 'Sorry.'

And she tells me very clearly, very calmly, 'It's OK.'

'Your hair will grow back, *Steph*. And it can be you, me, *Izzy* and the baby,' he says in that tone as delicate as roses.

I expect her to flinch, but Mum's voice is a fossil and Daniel hears it, sees it too, how she's unearthed this part of her that's been buried for years. 'There won't be a baby, Daniel.'

'You won't get away with it, you know.' His thorns come

out, but Mum's bald head pushes closer to the sky. He's an arm's length away now, his hand reaching for Mum's neck, Mum's ear, Mum's scalp, his eyes narrowing when she doesn't buckle under the nasty promise his fingers circle in figures of eight on her skin. 'Where's my pretty little girl gone, Stephanie?'

And then comes the flash. The flash of our lives since we met him. The flash of him on my mum and his fingers in her nose and his elbows in her stomach and his words constantly streaming in her head. The flash of his gifts and his promises and his shining-armour rescues and his tear-stained pleas. The flash of him pulling on her hair on her pretty little head. And as I push his arm away from her, she reaches into her bag and grabs the hairspray he'd insisted she carry everywhere, and as I raise my foot to his groin, she aims for his eyes. And even though we're not quite in sync, we make it work because together we move faster, stronger than if we were alone.

And when he falls to his knees with his face in his hands, we stand over him, looking back at where we've come from, at this ripple we've made in the water and at his other, bigger ripples we've survived.

'You hear that?' Mum says, holding my hand steady as the sound of sirens travels hard down the riverbank.

Daniel looks up, eyes squinting with the hairspray and the glare of the sun.

'That's the sound of an ending,' she says, but it feels like a beginning to me.

FIFTY-FIVE

We told them, the police. We answered their questions and made our statements and were told it could go to court, and the 'could' was a punch as hard as any of Daniel's. But we know. We know what happened. We know what he did. We know how it both ended and began by the river that cuts up and connects things. And we know too how hard it is to prove. Because the police told us, and Elizabeth told us, and Kate told us, and the internet told us, and the newspapers told us, and so we know.

But we'll try.

Mum was Superwoman in that battle with Daniel, but when she lies down on the bed at the clinic, she looks mortal, like invisible nettles are binding their stems around her skin. Her goosebumped arms run into fidgeting fingers, her eyes determinedly open as the nurse rubs a gel on her belly. And I'm sure she'll turn away from the screen where a black-and-white cashew nut is tethered to her insides, but she looks at the thing that's not a cashew nut, that's something else. And even though nothing hurts yet, not in her body anyway, I wish I could take away her pain.

'Yes, you're pregnant.' The nurse's voice is careful and kind and used to this. 'Eight weeks.'

Mum nods.

I help her get into Kate's car even though she says, 'I'm fine, Iz. Nothing will happen until after the second pill.'

But I have this need to be close to her, to have my hands where she might need them to hold her up.

We watch a movie when we get back to the refuge. Eat popcorn. And though we're not *not* saying anything, *Finding Nemo* is a distraction from the waiting, and when Nemo is found, so too is Mum's voice when she wriggles out of the hug I have her in and turns to face me.

'It *is* a loss, you know.' Her voice is a flag at half mast. 'If I'd had it –' we don't call it "the baby" now that we know it won't be – 'it may have been OK. I may have loved it. But I love you so much already, Izzy. And I'm just beginning to love me again too. That's what I'm protecting. I'm protecting us.'

I'm not allowed to go into the second appointment, so I give Mum my Jar of Sunshine to take in her bag.

She tells me afterwards that she held it as they gave her that second pill, that she squeezed on the glass and pictured my face when she'd put me to bed on those nights before Daniel, those yellow beads still on their strings around my neck as she read me a story, how I'd press my nose up against the glass of my bedroom window and say goodnight to our destination moon. 'That's what you taught me, Izzy,' she says, her voice tired from the disrupted sleep because of the cramping, 'with your sunshine and your moon: you taught me to always look up for the sky. There's so much hope up there.'

For a few days we are both quieter. And it's not like we wear black or say prayers, but we *are* mourning. Not just *it*. We're mourning the other losses too. We don't say it, not out loud, but we know. We know there are minutes and hours and days and weeks we can't get back. We know there are memories as permanent as Mum's scars. We know there are things we will do because of the things he did, but we know too that we will keep our noses pressed to the window always looking up for the sky.

A few weeks pass.

I talk to Grace.

I talk to Harry and kiss him too – long, slow kisses, which become something more urgent sometimes, but we wait and scull and imagine.

I talk to Mum about Daniel, about Harry. I even talk to her about Jacob.

'When Grace told me what he did…' she says.

I swear this is the moment she'll tell me about her disappointment but no.

'I'm so sorry,' she tells me.

'*You're* sorry? Mum, I'm the one who's sorry.'

'Why?' she says, and I don't understand the question, because it's obvious, isn't it?

'Because…'

She looks at me, like, *how did you get to be this big?* 'You have nothing to be sorry for, Izzy. That boy on the other hand…That's why I had to tell the college. I had to stop him from hurting you. Do you see?'

'But I…'

'You what?'

'Grace says it was…' But it can't be true, can it? What Grace says *it* was? Because I walked into his room, didn't I? I lay down on his bed, didn't I? I stayed quiet, didn't I? I let it happen, didn't I?

Didn't I?

'Grace is right,' Mum says. And her voice is this weird mix of dynamite and grief.

'I could have left.'

'So could I,' she says. 'In theory.'

'Yeah, but Daniel made it so you couldn't.'

'Exactly.' And her eyes are like, *you see what I'm getting at, Izzy?*

And I do but...

'Cheese?' She's making us a sandwich, and she says this too like it's the same kind of *no big deal*: 'We could go to the police.'

But the thought of saying everything aloud...

I write him, Jacob, a letter until my hand aches. I tell him how it felt, what he did to me, what he did to all of us with his phone and his pressure and his take, take, take. Grace will pass it on for me; I don't imagine she'll be asked to pass me a reply.

But you never know.

When autumn comes, Mum and I listen to *Desert Island Discs* in our new flat, on two green charity-shop chairs, which we push up opposite each other, so they make an island in the room.

The castaway is a geologist who says how your senses are dulled in Antarctica. How the mass of blue and white does something to your eyes, and the lack of noise does something to your ears, and all that cold deadens your smell and your taste. It's only when you go home that your senses reawaken and your awareness of your own body becomes whole again.

Mum and I sit in our fusty green chairs listening, seeing, tasting, smelling, touching.

Whole.

FIFTY-SIX

No more sneaking out on the water at 6.00 A.M. I'm a legit sculler now. With a coach and lessons and everything. Full access to the club, with a huge room full of things they say are called sweep boats and sculling boats and oars and blades, but to me they're all just keys. Because when I'm out on the water, it feels like I've unlocked another world.

They've even let me out on my own. Just me in charge on the river, this instructor Dean calling from the jetty to remember my wrists, watch my legs, shoulders down, back strong, and I'm doing well, he says, until, along with the rest of life beyond the water, he disappears. Because I have this moment when the pushing and the pulling and the arms and the thighs are connected to the boat with invisible threads of gold, when my body has this rhythm that's all the music of my desert island and all the power of my broken pieces. This moment when the riverbanks drop away, and I could be anywhere. This moment when I choose to be here, on my own, moving without watching where I'm going, trusting my body to do its thing. Eyes on the water, eyes on the sky.

'She's amazing,' Harry says to Grace and Nell when we meet up with them in London. 'She's so elegant on the river.'

And it's a good job Nell's so Zen because Grace starts choking and spatters her with wine.

'Elegant? Izzy?' But her voice is a happy place, and her smile is a bolt of sunshine as we toast to my grace on the water and then again to my Grace in the bar.

'I goddamn miss you,' she says when it's time to say goodbye.

'I goddamn miss you too,' I tell her, and she gives me a thumbs up, stumbling into Nell's shoulder as they make their way down into the Tube.

'Ready?' Harry's talking about the walk back to the hotel, but I get the sense he's talking about The Other Thing too.

When we get to our room, it's not the penthouse, but it's the closest to the clouds I've ever been.

'Come here.' And I reach out to Harry, who slips an arm around my shoulder as we take in the view. 'It's so huge.'

'Well, thanks, but we haven't even started yet – you wait till we really get going.'

'Yeah right.' My elbow's soft into his side. 'I'm sure your Hobnob is enormous, Harry, but I was talking about the sky.'

'Both are pretty impressive.' And his laugh is full of nerves and excitement and *this will be OK*.

Which it is and then it isn't. Because when we lay down, his lips are on my lips and his hands are everywhere I've said they can be. And it feels so good, more than good even, but then it begins to feel fast, and I sense it, that shift when I run the risk of drifting, of lying back and letting it happen instead of it being something I've said yes to.

'Stop,' I say, kind of quiet, but I say it. I definitely say it.

And he does. Stop, I mean.

With a comical rearrangement of his boxers, Harry sits up, pours us some water and suggests we eat Hobnobs while listening to *Desert Island Discs*. 'My thing plus your thing equals our thing.'

We scroll through the episodes, and there's this one that must have aired in the heights of our leaving Daniel because I missed it.

'I've heard her talk before,' Harry says, 'The COO of Facebook. She's cool.'

We turn off the lights, crawl beneath the covers and press *play*.

The castaway's voice is strength and survival and a determination to make light in the dark.

'You seriously reckon that's true?' Harry asks, when she suggests girls are told not to take charge from an early age and at the same time boys are told that they must.

'Dunno,' I say, as he wraps his biscuit-crumbed hand around mine. 'Probably.'

All those times I've gone with the flow instead of using my voice – how, at some point, it became lost property.

The castaway's husband died of a heart attack when he was just forty-seven. Her voice when she describes it sounds like the end of the world. But then, in her friends and her children, and in her realisation that she deserves better than to feel unhappy for the rest of her life, she sounds like hope.

It's up there with the best of them, this *Desert Island Discs* episode, because she's open and honest. And her music – while looking backwards, it carries her forward too.

'You OK?' Harry asks when we're done with the island, turning on a lamp so he can see my face.

And I realise I am. OK, I mean. Not I'll-never-think-about-Daniel-or-Jacob kind of OK. But definitely I-deserve-not-to-be-unhappy OK. Because, for all the listening to castaways and compiling my own playlists, I don't want to be stranded, not now. I want to be here. With Harry. I want to come out of the cold and not feel guilty or dirty when all the parts of me start coming alive.

'Yes. And everything you've organised – the seeing Grace, the hotel, you – it's all perfect,' I say. And though it's not exactly booming, my voice is the beginning of something new. 'And I really want to have sex with you, Harry, honestly I do. And I will but —'

'So you're not ready?' Harry's voice is like, *this is cool, Izzy. All of this is cool.*

'Not just yet,' I say. 'No.' And the word is the most positive negative.

'Then we'll wait,' Harry says, just like that. His smile no less broad, his hold no less safe. His love no less.

But more.

FIFTY-SEVEN

I told Grace she didn't need to come. But...

'Just try and *goddamn* stop me,' she says now, using my headrest to pull herself up from the back seat so she can smother my cheek with a kiss.

'Do I look all right?'

And I know what she probably wants to say is: '*It shouldn't matter what you look like – they shouldn't be interested in how you dress. All that shit should be irrelevant.*' But all she actually says is: 'Fuckin' perfect, Izzy. You're literally fuckin' perfect.'

Mum nods, totally not bothered by the swears because *they're* not the words that matter. Not today.

The click of Grace's seat belt is the start of a ticking clock.

The car is filled with Sunday's *Desert Island Discs*. And Grace is all 'Shit, shit', trying to stop the podcast on her phone when the castaway starts talking about how she found her mum knocked out by her father on the kitchen floor. 'Shit.' Grace's fingers are flustering again, and when I turn around, she looks surprised by my grin.

'Let's listen.'

Grace shrugs her shoulders, hits *play*.

She sounds happy, the guest. Fulfilled. In wonder at what she's achieved. And it doesn't make any of the pain she went through any less significant; it doesn't mean the screams she heard downstairs or the blood she saw on her mother's face don't count. They happened. And although they did, she survived. And right now she's totally destination moon.

When we get there, both of them, my mum and my best friend, take me by the hand as we walk in. My stabilisers. And it's just like I remember: I feel braver, more able to try this out with them here.

I made a call, see. Not to the police, not yet. But to something Mum found online: Independent Sexual Violence Advisers. And it was easier to read it than to hear it when I phoned them, so I thrust my mobile at Mum and she asked, in this voice that acted like my buffer, absorbing some of the shock that keeps on coming, if there was someone I could speak with.

'My daughter was raped,' she said.

And *I* may not have said anything, not then, but I kept my eyes open, my head up, and that's a start, right?

So Mum spoke, and we agreed that I'd come in. That there'd be someone I could talk to. Not the police, not yet. But someone who will listen. 'When you're able to talk,' Mum said.

She's a counsellor, I guess, this woman who comes to meet me in reception, this woman who smiles at me and Mum and Grace, but at me mostly. This woman who tells them there's a cafe down the road if they want to grab a coffee, who nods, like, *I get it*, when Mum says they'll stay in the waiting room if that's OK.

She tells me her name, this woman, and although I nod, I don't remember it, even though she remembers mine and uses it often, like it's important, like that's the word in the room with the most meaning. Like I'm way more Izzy than I am anything else.

'Would you like to talk to me about what happened?' she asks.

'Yes,' I say.

And the word is an expanding universe.

And my voice?

Well, my voice is the goddamn Big Bang.

ACKNOWLEDGEMENTS

If you want to write stories, it helps to be raised on magic. On birthdays when I was a kid, my dad would pull Sindy dolls from hats and make the names of playing cards appear from ash rubbed into his skin. He's since offered to tell me how it was done but I already know. He, like the five other adults – Mum, Pam, Phil, Mel and Graham – who raised my friends and me on The Green, were of another world. A world in which the twelve of us came together on the perfectly named (albeit imperfectly spelt) Galaxie Road in Portsmouth, where dens, trees, fireworks, pantomimes, picnics, Christmases and New Year's Eves were imbued with a celestial quality which filled me with a cocky kind of certainty that anything and everything can be magical. And so, if anything and everything can be magical surely anything and everything can be possible too. While Izzy's experience with Jacob and Daniel is in direct contrast to my own experience on The Green, the writing of it is a direct consequence of all the love I was given there. I am so very lucky. Thank you, you wonderful six.

If you want to write stories, it helps to be raised on books. Thanks to Mum I read widely and indiscriminately. Summers were a mix of Thomas Hardy's *Tess of the D'Urbervilles* and Jackie Collins' *Hollywood Wives*, though our favourites were never without a woman on a discovery of her own self-worth.

So thanks, Mum, for the books, the life lessons and the reading of almost every word I've written. And for saying it's good even when it probably isn't. My desire to write strong female characters stems, no doubt, from the fact that I was brought up by one. I love you millipons.

If you want to write stories, it helps to be raised with guts. Thanks, Dad, for showing me it's worth taking that leap of faith. Emigrating to Canada and training to be a ski instructor in your sixties is no mean feat. Obviously, I miss you, but I'm so proud of, and inspired by, you taking your dream and running with it. #SkiInstructorOfTheYearForever

If you want to write stories, it helps to be raised with grit. Thanks to Karl for instilling resilience in the way only a brother can. By pinning me down and drooling over my face until your saliva was almost touching my nose. Thanks for sucking it back up again before it did. And for making me laugh, even when it was your spit that almost made me cry. You taught me to see the funny side.

If you want to write stories, it helps to be raised on fairy tale. Big thanks to my very own fairy godmother Teresa Kwasny for a lifetime of magical experiences to fuel my writerly brain.

If you want to write stories, magic, books, guts, grit and fairy tale all help, but as the brilliant writer and all-round super woman Stella Duffy repeatedly told me, there is actually only one solution. Write The Fucking Book. Thanks, Stella. The Arvon retreat with you and Shelley got me going but your wise words, now my mantra (#WTFB), got me to the end.

Writing stories is hard. I often feel not only is what I'm writing rubbish, but that I am pretty useless too. I'm not alone. So huge thanks to all my stoic writer friends, who not only understand this feeling but manage to hoik me *and* my work out of the doldrums with their edits, their ideas and their cake.

Sue Bassett, our rope now stretches 243 miles but is, I think, all the stronger for it. You are rope and rock and ally. And – are you ready for this? – for someone who doesn't believe in fate, I actually think, what with Fun Palaces and book swaps and Nanowrimo, our friendship was genuinely meant to be.

Sandra Dingwall. Says it like it is. One of *the* most important traits when critiquing. Even if it does make me a little scared, afterwards I'm always grateful. Cheers for your wise and sweary words, which have not only made a huge difference to my books but to my life in Shropshire.

And to my broader writing groups, thanks for putting up with my wobbly voiced readings. You are such a great source of advice, ideas and, well, wine.

I'm massively grateful to all those who read early drafts. Megan Mackenzie, who also answers my random texts about teenagers, Koshesai Fundira, Amy Haslam, Toria Lyle and Josie Phillips.

Special thanks to everyone on the writer's retreat at Chez Castillon. Izzy would never have made it on to the river if it wasn't for you. And Julie Cohen, you forced me to make shit happen. And then some more shit. Followed by a little more to boot. Thank you for encouraging me to really put Izzy through it.

Big thanks to my agent Hannah Sheppard, who, when asking to meet me, proved magic happens when you're a grownup too. Your editorial guidance has been invaluable, as has your ability to humour me when – in moments of despair – I genuinely believed space hopper-shaped cookies could be the answer.

The writing process is filled with self-doubt and a fair bit of crying. After meeting my publishers for the first time, I walked to the station, got on the train and promptly burst into tears. This time, happy ones. Shadi Doostdar, Gill Evans, Harriet Wade, Aimee Oliver-Powell, Kate Bland, Molly Scull and Laura McFarlane, thanks so so much for believing in Izzy. And in me. Gill, your edits were all spot on, I might – if I were pushing a theme here – go as far as to say they worked like magic. (Ps. They did.)

And to the rest of the team at Rock the Boat, thank you for turning my story into an actual real-life, hold-it-in-your-hands and maybe-even-kiss-it book. That right there is wizardry.

Cheers to Dean Bishton at Pengwern Boat Club for taking me out on the river, to Claire Evans at Cafcass and to Sasha, for sharing your own experience of domestic abuse. I'm so happy that, like Izzy, you are able to use your voice.

To my funny, kind, superstar children, Monty and Dolly. I hope your voices, which are these days filled with funfair, moxie and magic, continue to be loud and strong and filled with your own self-worth. Because you are worth everything. I love you more than hot chocolate. Fact.

Thanks to *Game of Thrones* and Netflix for providing my husband with entertainment so he didn't so much mind the evenings *I* spent writing and *he* spent alone.

And Phil. It is not an exaggeration to say I couldn't have done this without you. There are so many reasons why. From our first not-date when I dribbled orange juice through my nose, you retained a faith in me so absolute it overcame heart-aches, foreign departures and, even, an exercise ball popped in wild and frustrated fury. You gave me time and space. You gave me a desk. You even gave me a room of one's own. Most importantly, you gave me love. When I said I wanted to open a stationery shop and you said no, I called you a dream smasher. What I realise now is that you were never smashing my dream but doing your utmost to ensure that the real one – this one! – came true. And that, MDH, is the very best magic of all.

HELP AND SUPPORT (UK)

British Pregnancy Advisory Service
www.bpas.org
03457 30 40 30
Help and support for unplanned pregnancy and abortion.

Brook
www.brook.org.uk
Confidential information and support regarding sexual health, sexual wellbeing and contraception for people under twenty-five.

Childline
www.childline.org.uk
0800 1111
Support for young people, no matter what they're going through.

Disrespect Nobody
www.disrespectnobody.co.uk
Information and support on relationship abuse, sexting, consent, rape, porn and harassment.

Jewish Women's Aid

www.jwa.org.uk
Domestic abuse helpline: 0808 801 0500
Sexual violence support: 0808 801 0656
Support for Jewish women and children affected by domestic and sexual violence.

Men's Advice Line

www.mensadviceline.org.uk
0808 801 0327
Advice and support for men experiencing domestic violence and abuse.

Nour Domestic Violence Support

www.nour-dv.org.uk
Provides access to professional and legal Islamic advisors who are able to offer psychological support and appropriate counselling to victims of domestic violence.

Rape Crisis England & Wales

www.rapecrisis.org.uk
0808 802 9999
Independent specialist support services for women and girls who have experienced child sexual abuse, rape or any kind of sexual violence at any time.

Refuge

www.refuge.org.uk
0808 2000 247

Freephone 24 Hour National Domestic Violence Helpline run in partnership between Women's Aid and Refuge.
Help for women and children experiencing domestic abuse.

Samaritans
www.samaritans.org
116 123
Whatever you're going through, Samaritans will listen.

Scarleteen
www.scarleteen.com
Inclusive support regarding sexuality and relationships for teens and young adults.

Survivors UK
www.survivorsuk.org
Information and support for boys and men who have been raped or sexually abused.

Welsh Women's Aid
www.welshwomensaid.org.uk
0808 80 10 800

Women's Aid
www.womensaid.org.uk
0808 2000 247
Freephone 24 Hour National Domestic Violence Helpline run in partnership between Women's Aid and Refuge.
Help for women and children experiencing domestic abuse.

HELP AND SUPPORT (US)

RAINN (Rape, Abuse & Incest National Network)
online.rainn.org
National Sexual Assault Hotline: 800-656-HOPE (4673)
The largest anti-sexual violence organisation in the United
States of America.

End Rape On Campus
endrapeoncampus.org
Works to end campus sexual violence by supporting survivors, education and policy reform.

FORGE
forge-forward.org
A national transgender anti-violence organisation helping
transgender, gender nonconforming and gender nonbinary
survivors of sexual assault.

1in6
1in6.org
Support for male victims of unwanted sexual experiences,
sexual abuse and sexual violence.

National Sexual Violence Resource Center

nsvrc.org

A national information and resource organisation that works with the Centers for Disease Control and Prevention to collect and share resources with people and organisations trying to understand and eliminate sexual violence.

Safe Horizon

safehorizon.org

Offers resources to survivors of human trafficking, child abuse, stalking, youth homelessness and domestic violence.

The Trevor Project

thetrevorproject.org

1-866-488-7386

Crisis intervention and suicide prevention for LGBTQ+ youth, offering a hotline (phone, text and online chat), and educational resources for family and allies.

Planned Parenthood

plannedparenthood.org

Provides vital reproductive health care, sex education and information.

QUESTIONS FOR DISCUSSION

1. Why does Max feel unable to speak out against Jacob at the start of the novel? Is his silence comparable to Izzy's?

2. On page 94, Izzy describes a moment of realisation: 'I guess that's when I first realised how small our lives are... how people rarely look beyond their horizon.' (p.94) Do you think this realisation is important to the rest of the narrative? Is Izzy also guilty of not being able to see beyond her horizon?

3. Do Steph and Grace have some culpability in Izzy's unhappiness? What does the novel teach us about what it means to be a good person?

4. Silence is one of the novel's major themes. Is there a relationship between silence and shame?

5. When Izzy's mum Steph went back to Daniel the first time, Izzy lost her sense of safety. Do you agree with Izzy that: 'It's like riding a bike, I guess, that ability to feel safe again: all you need is the vehicle and your body remembers the rest.'? (p. 106) Do you think she feels safe again by the end of the novel?

6. Jacob and Daniel both inflict physical harm on Izzy and Steph. Must violence be overt to cause harm? What do you understand by the word coercion?

7. To what extent does love play a role in the book?

8. There is a gap between what Izzy feels and what she does. Why do you think this is? Is there always a conflict between our thoughts and our actions?

9. 'I hadn't known she was in me, that girl who won't stand for it, that girl who won't sit quietly on the sidelines while those boys flaunt their god-given 'right' to say and do what they want with our bodies. Where's she been all these years?' (p.149) Why does Izzy decide now that she will no longer be silenced? Do you think this is the first time she realises she has been mistreated?

10. In light of Izzy's story, what do you understand by consent? Should consent be taught in schools?